Pilates

Creating the body you want

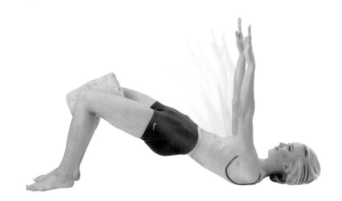

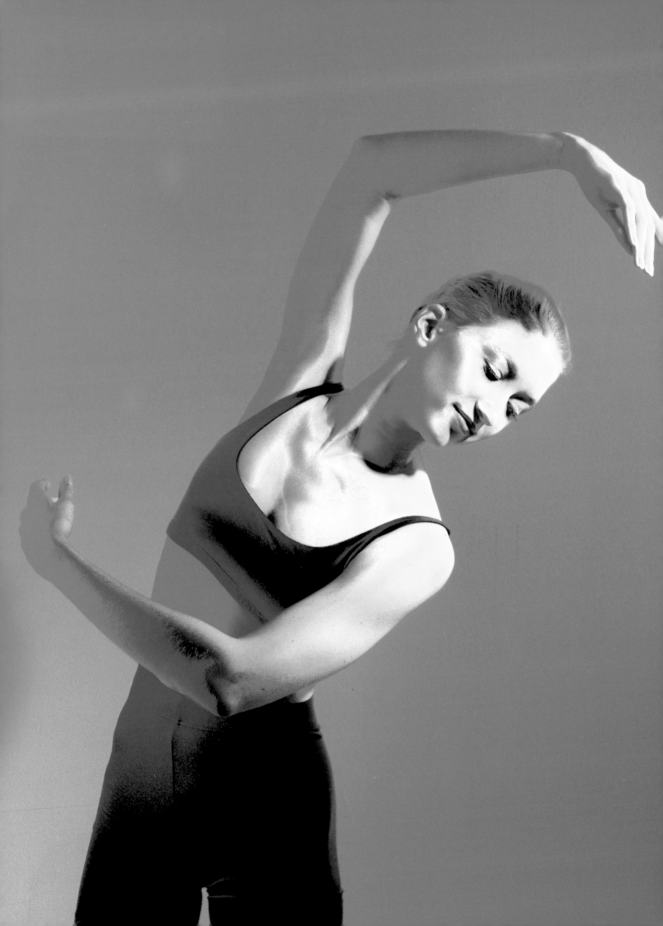

Pilates

Creating the body you want

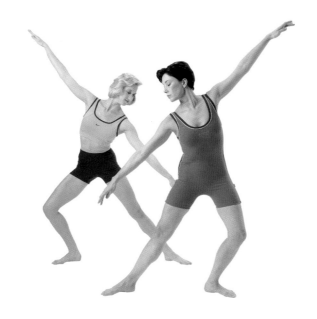

Anna Selby & Alan Herdman

Gaia Books

A Gaia Original

Books from Gaia celebrate the vision of Gaia, the self-sustaining living Earth, and seek to help readers live in greater personal and planetary harmony.

Designer	Phil Gamble
Editors	Helena Petre, Camilla Davis
Photography	Paul Forrester, Andy Rumball
Managing Editor	Pip Morgan
Production	Lyn Kirby
Direction	Patrick Nugent

CAUTION
The techniques, ideas and suggestions in this book are to be used at the reader's sole discretion and risk. Always observe the cautions given, and consult a doctor if in doubt about a medical condition.

 ® This is a Registered Trade Mark of Gaia Books

Copyright © 2005 Gaia Books
an imprint of Octopus Publishing Group Ltd
2–4 Heron Quays, London, E14 4JP

First published in the United Kingdom in 1999 by
Gaia Books Ltd

ISBN 1-85675-258-5
EAN 9781856752589

A catalogue record of this book is available from the British Library.

Printed and bound in China
10 9 8 7 6 5 4 3 2 1

How to use this book

This book has been constructed as a progressive course. Your programme starts with a self-assessment to help you identify your strengths and weaknesses, and locate important and often forgotten muscles. It is a good idea to go back to these self-assessment exercises over the weeks to come to see how you have changed – always an uplifting experience.

The warm-up that starts on page 48 is common to all levels – do it at the start of every session to help you focus and become body-aware before you go on to the more complex movements that follow. Each level works every part of your body but you will, of course, find that some parts of you are stronger or more flexible than others. However, it is best to be able to do all of the exercises in each level comfortably before going on to the next. Within each level some exercises are harder than others, so leave ones such as the advanced abdominals in level three until you are really strong. It is particularly important to build up the 'girdle of strength', the pelvic and abdominal support for the whole body, gradually, so that you can take on more difficult movements safely. If your abdominal muscles bulge or quiver, stop! This is a warning that they aren't strong enough yet to perform the exercise. In this case, do fewer repetitions or try not to go so far.

The number of repetitions is specified in each exercise. Don't be tempted to do more – it is quality and precision that count in Pilates technique, not quantity. Ideally, aim for three sessions a week with a rest day between each one.

The exercises in this book are all non-aerobic and, to supplement them, we recommend regular aerobic exercise. Brisk walking is easy to incorporate into your daily routine, and swimming and cycling are also ideal. Running or jogging, however, are all too likely to cause injury, notably to knees and backs, particularly if you run on a hard surface, such as a pavement. Try to take two or three 20-minute exercise periods each week, choosing exercise that leaves you slightly out of breath.

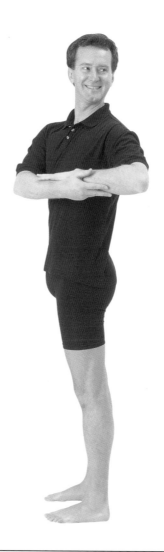

Contents

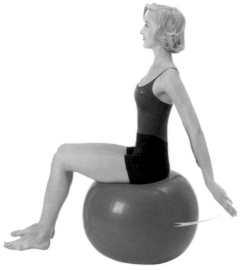

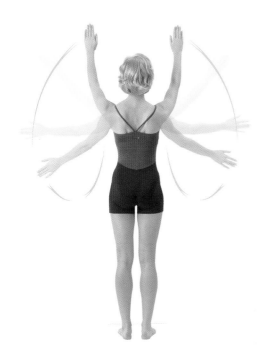

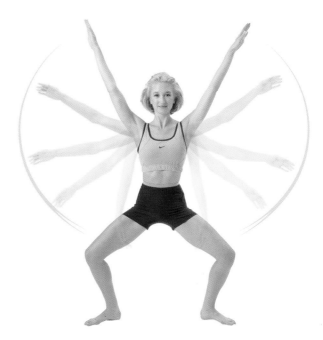

Foreword

I have been practising the Pilates' exercising technique at Alan's studio for about seventeen years. I have also been 'floored' and 'at it' in hotel rooms all over the world. Pilates exercises are precisely the kind I need and like. One doesn't have to dance about and 'burn', one merely tones all the muscles in the body. So many of the wonderful new exercise routines introduced these days are found to be injurious from various points of view a year or two later.

Apart from a general feeling of well-being created by doing Pilates exercises, I find them invaluable in keeping me out of the osteopath's hands. I have a back problem exacerbated by the practice of judo on the cement studio floor during the Avengers, and provided the muscles in my back are kept strong and flexible, I find my vertebrae remain exactly where they should be.

I wrote a book a couple of years ago about how to stay vigorous, stylish and groomed, and one of the most vital chapters involved Pilates exercises. Indeed it includes a jolly picture of Alan and me as he was good enough to help me with all the appropriate names for the muscles. I remember saying in the book that all that one needed to exercise efficiently at home was a kitchen chair, a cushion, a book, a couple of cans of soup and a small towel. That's what's so wonderful about Pilates exercises – you need no expensive equipment and you can get on with it anywhere – well almost anywhere.

Alan is a wonderful instructor – and quite severe. There is no point in vaguely waltzing through exercises, one must concentrate and be sure that one achieves the object of the exercise. A shorter period of time with the job done thoroughly is worth more than twice the time rushed and inefficiently performed.

Before I start my exercises I often think 'Oh gawd' but at the end I'm upright, walking tall and feeling marvellous and vibrant (a favourite word of my old stablemate, Patrick Macnee).

I can leave you in Alan's hands with total confidence. Go to it and it is one decision you will have made in life – and keep to – that you will never regret.

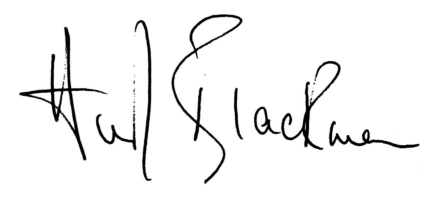

Honor Blackman

About the authors

Anna Selby has been involved in many forms of dance and exercise, including ballet, Martha Graham technique, yoga and tai chi. However, her first interest was the Pilates technique, and in 1985 her *Woman's Workout Book* was the first book in the UK to include the subject. She has subsequently written nine more books, mostly on exercise and health, including aromatherapy and Chinese herbal medicine. Having been a features reporter for BBC radio's immensely popular *Woman's Hour*, she is now a freelance feature writer for a variety of UK newspapers and magazines, including *The Times*, *The Daily Telegraph*, *Evening Standard*, and *Harpers & Queen*.

Alan Herdman is the leading practitioner of Pilates technique in the UK. Having learned the method in New York, he introduced it to London in 1970, and set up the first Pilates studio in England. His previous training was with London Contemporary Dance in Martha Graham technique. He was also trained as a teacher in Laban Dance Drama. As well as his London studio, he has established several others around the world, including in Sweden and Israel. As a teacher trainer, he has passed on his knowledge and expertise to many Pilates teachers, as well as to dancers of the English National Ballet, the London School of Contemporary Dance, the Houston Ballet and Israel's Bat-Dor Dance Company. He also works with the Royal Academy of Dance, the English National Ballet School and Company, and Elmhurst Ballet School, and is a guest teacher every year in Japan and the US.

Introduction

Joseph Pilates was fond of pointing out that he had invented a technique that was 50 years ahead of its time.

Given its enormous popularity now, we can only concur. It has spread from a single studio in New York frequented by professional dancers to a technique with worldwide appeal practised by people from every age group and background.

The reasons for such success are rooted in the fact that, quite simply, it works. After the endless exercise fads of recent decades, this technique has emerged as the one most likely to give you the body you want in the safest possible way.

Most forms of sport and exercise concentrate on the larger, stronger muscles and, as these get stronger and bulkier, the smaller weaker muscles are forgotten. In Pilates technique, however, these weaker muscles – often ones that many people are not even aware of – are strengthened, while the larger muscles become increasingly toned and sleek, creating a balanced, lithe, integrated body. Locating these smaller muscles and learning how to use them requires a great deal of concentration, control and precision – and, for this reason, Pilates technique is commonly referred to as 'thinking exercise'. It requires an unusual synchronicity of mind and body and this, in turn, results in a sense of wholeness and integration more commonly associated with eastern meditative and movement techniques.

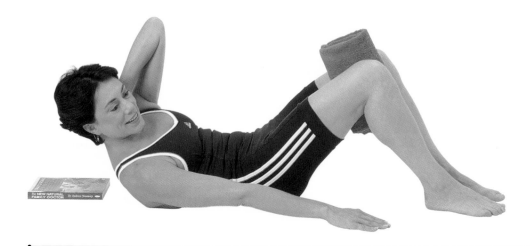

Concentration is one of the six basic principles of Pilates technique – reflected in Joseph Pilates' own favourite quotation from the poet Schiller, 'It is the mind itself that builds the body.' The other basic principles are breathing, control, centring, flowing movement and precision. Because the exercises are so controlled, they are very safe – the technique is ideal, for instance, for those in rehabilitation after an accident. It is also perfect for any age – as is made evident by the numerous 70-year-olds in Alan Herdman's London studio.

This is the technique in which you finally get to know your own body. As you learn through the exercises how to use Pilates properly, your posture improves, your muscles become more toned, your joints more mobile and your body shape becomes more balanced, poised and elongated. This is achieved not by endless repetitions of mind-numbingly boring exercises, but by minimal movements that use controlled muscles rather than momentum. At first it may seem that little is happening, especially if you are used to aerobic classes or gyms where you lift heavy weights. However, to be able to use your body correctly, you have to become aware of it as an integrated entity – so many of the early exercises in this book are about locating forgotten muscles and learning how to move your body to achieve the best possible results.

By working your way through the levels in this book, you can expect to achieve the body you have always wanted. You may not necessarily lose weight – muscles weigh more than fat – but you will flatten your stomach, tone and elongate your limbs, lift your buttocks and have the poise and elegance of a dancer. Best of all, the lessons learned here spill over into everyday life, so even the most routine activities – sitting, walking or standing – become infused with grace and balance.

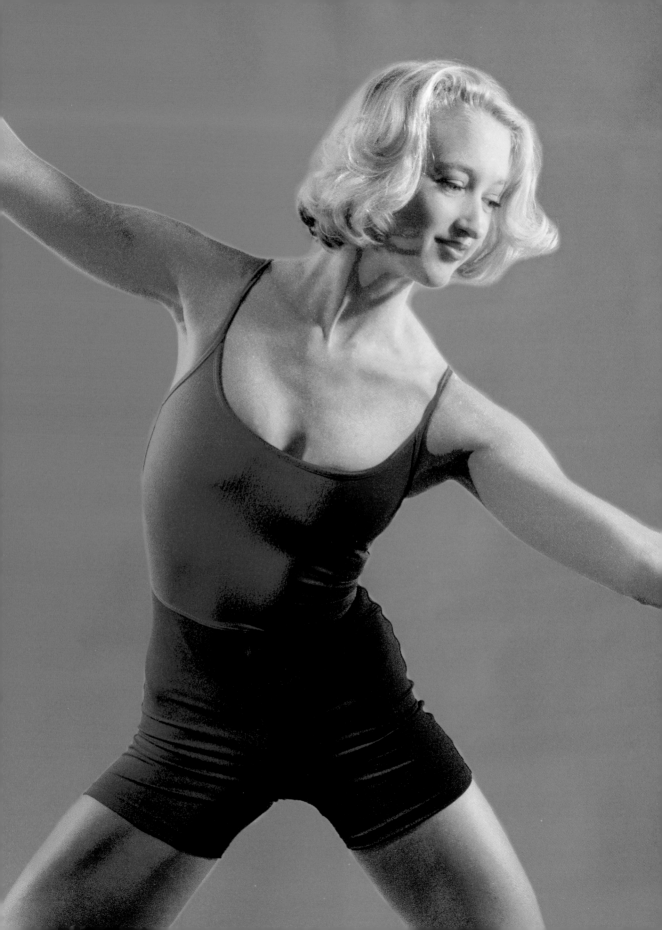

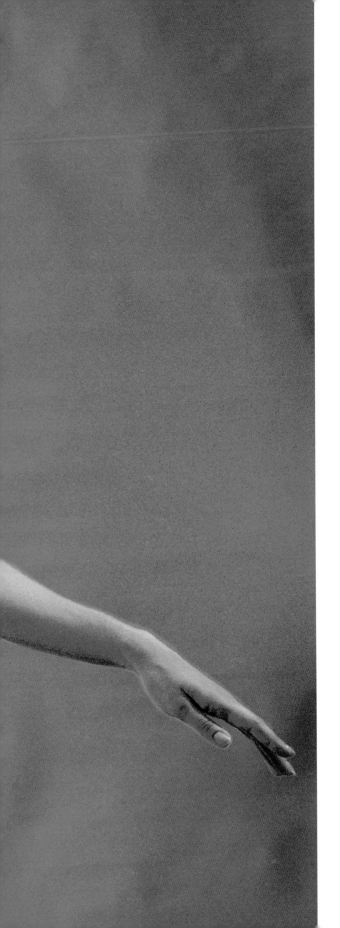

Chapter One

The Birth of Pilates Technique

Joseph Hubertus Pilates was born in 1880 near Düsseldorf in Germany. He was a frail child, regarded as prone to tuberculosis.

However, so determined was he to improve his physical condition, that instead of being limited by it, he worked relentlessly at body-building and conditioning until, by the age of fourteen, he was posing as a model for anatomical drawings. He went on to become a keen sportsman in various fields: he was a gymnast, a skier, a diver, a boxer – even a circus performer. In 1912, he left his native Germany for England where he became a professional boxer and taught self-defence to detectives at Scotland Yard.

When the First World War broke out, two years after Joseph Pilates move from Germany to Britain, the British authorities interned him as a German national, and he decided to use his enforced 'leisure' to develop his ideas about health and physical fitness. His influences were wide-ranging, to say the least, embracing everything from yoga to the study of animal movements. He instructed his fellow internees in his evolving techniques and claimed that, because of this, not one of them died in the influenza epidemic of 1918.

After the war he returned to Germany and worked with most of the pioneers of movement technique but most closely with Rudolf von Laban, the creator of the form of dance notation widely used today. At the same time, Joseph

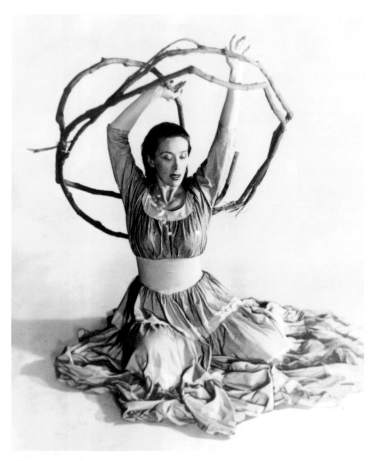

MARTHA GRAHAM
American choreographer, dancer, teacher and pioneer of 'modern dance', as she appears in *Salem Shore* (c.1924).

Pilates was working as a trainer for the Hamburg police force. However, he did not stay in Germany long. In 1923, he left for New York to set up his first studio with his wife Clara.

Joseph Pilates' method was an immediate success in America, particularly amongst dancers – Martha Graham and George Balanchine were early converts. Dancers, necessarily prone to injury, soon discovered that rehabilitation using Pilates exercises led to a swifter recovery – and this at a time when the therapeutic effects of immediate rehabilitation had not been recognised. However, during his internment, Joseph Pilates had worked for a while as a nurse. In this capacity, he had experimented with springs attached to hospital beds so that patients could begin to work on toning their muscles, even before they could get up.

Using springs as resistance again, Joseph Pilates designed the machine he called his 'universal reformer', a sliding, horizontal bed that can be used with up to four springs, according to the exercise and the strength of the individual. Nowadays, the descendant of the universal reformer is usually known as a plié machine and it is still central to the Pilates studio. Other machines were developed, and the exercise method grew and spread over the decades.

Alan Herdman introduced the method to Britain in the early 1970s after studying Pilates technique in New York with two of Joseph Pilates' foremost disciples, Bob Fitzgerald and Carola Trier, who were personally trained by Joseph Pilates. Alan's studio in London is now an internationally respected centre for the technique. Over the decades since Joseph Pilates set up his studio, his technique has been developed in a variety of ways. Some teachers have used a percussive, fast-paced method with effort coinciding with the in-breath. This tends to build bulky muscles at the expense of the less-developed ones. One of the most distinctive features of Alan Herdman's teaching is the focused breathing, where all effort is placed on the out-breath, leading both to a supremely balanced and poised body and a relaxed, focused mind. All movements are extremely slow and rhythmic, allowing weaker muscles to be located and well worked.

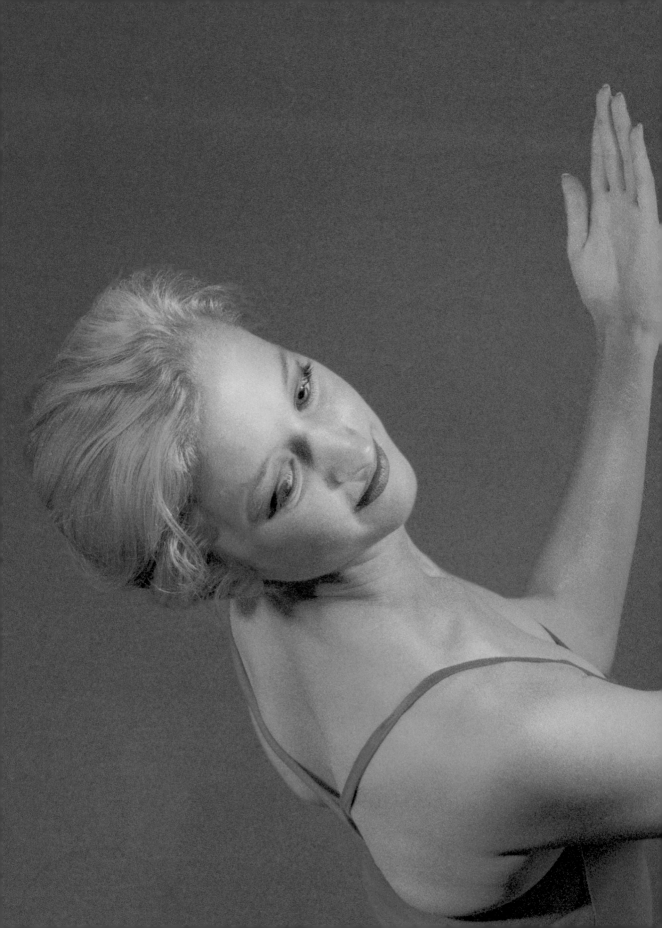

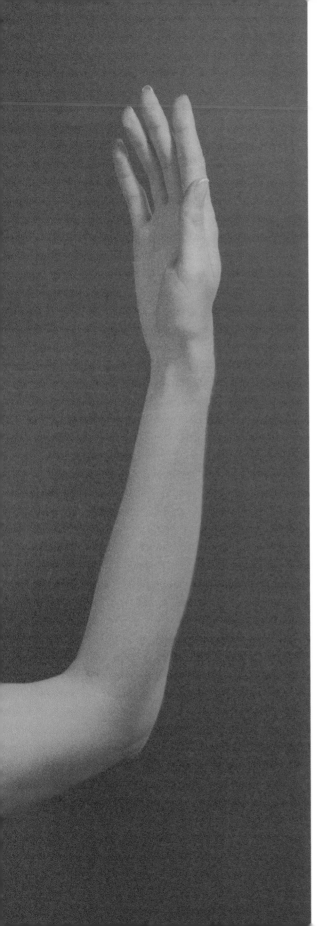

Chapter Two

Your Body Basics

. . . .

*Before you begin to exercise,
take time to assess your own
body. We all have bad habits of
posture and the ways we move
and it is vital to recognise and
correct these before you begin.*

*One of the most important aspects of Pilates
technique is that it starts with fundamentals –
posture and breathing – and all the exercises
build on these foundations. Body Basics
shows you how to assess your own posture
and breathing with simple exercises that use
either the floor or a mirror. Take time on these
basic assessments before you begin to
exercise – it will repay you tenfold when you
get started.*

Muscle groups of the body

In Pilates technique, you use your muscles in a very precise and focused way. The emphasis is on the quality of the movement, often with many muscles being used in synchronicity within any given exercise. Some of these are likely to be weak from under-use – so much so that they may be difficult to locate. These pages show where the main muscle groups are. For a further explanation of how to use them in Pilates technique, see the glossary on p. 139.

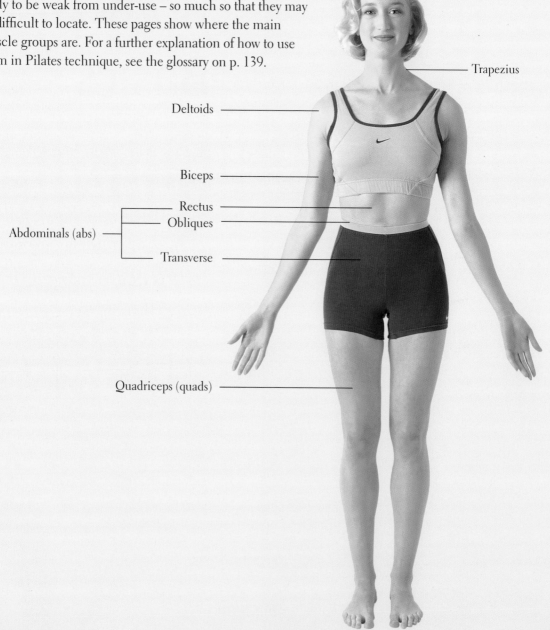

Trapezius

Deltoids

Biceps

Rectus

Obliques

Abdominals (abs)

Transverse

Quadriceps (quads)

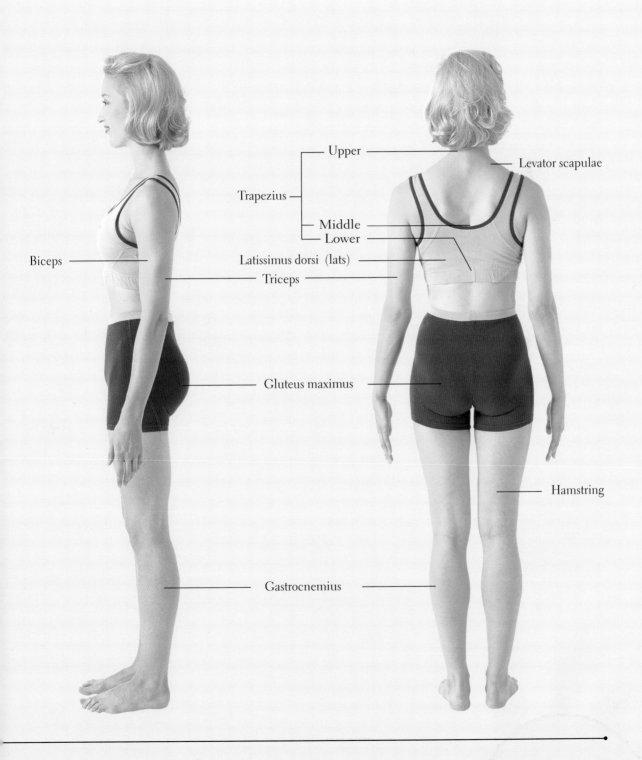

Upper

Levator scapulae

Trapezius

Middle

Lower

Biceps

Latissimus dorsi (lats)

Triceps

Gluteus maximus

Hamstring

Gastrocnemius

Good and bad posture

One of the great benefits of Pilates technique is the elongated posture you achieve, with the loose, graceful shape of a dancer. Beyond appearances, however, good posture is vital while you're exercising, and it helps you get the maximum benefit from your workout. If you don't hold on to your abdominal muscles while you exercise, you're in danger of straining your back, while moving your arms from tense neck and shoulders will only increase tension, and will probably give you a headache as well.

The photograph of bad posture (near right) may look somewhat exaggerated when compared with the photograph of good posture (far right), and you would be very unlucky to start off with all of the problems shown. However, it does indicate the most common postural faults, and it is a good idea to start your own assessment in front of a mirror, comparing your own body shape with the one shown here. Look both front and sideways on to the mirror and go through this checklist at your own pace.

Head and neck
Does your chin jut out or tilt upwards? If so, it is pulling your spine out of alignment and shortening the muscles in the back of the neck. We tend to forget that the back of the neck is the top of the spine and, by compressing it, the spine itself is put under pressure and distorted. To put your head and neck in the right position, look straight ahead, with your chin pulled very slightly backwards. Feel as if the top of your head is attached to a piece of string that is pulling it away from your body, lengthening out your neck and spine.

Shoulders and arms
These areas are often the seat of tension in the body and the cause of both bad posture and headaches. Look in the mirror to see if your shoulders and upper back roll forward. Perhaps they are pulled rigidly back, sergeant-major fashion, pushing out the breastbone. Are they even? One shoulder is often tensed and held higher than the other, simply as a result of habitually carrying bags on one side. Check the photographs

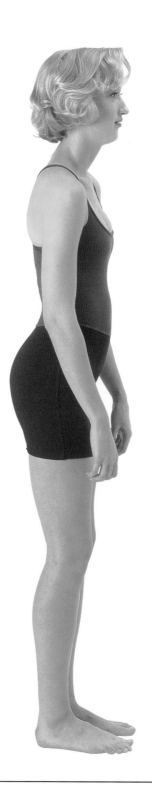

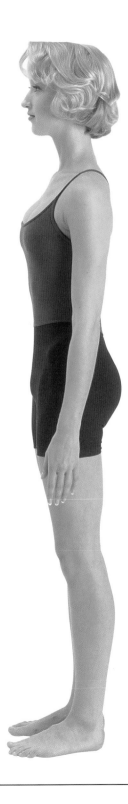

here and try to let your own shoulders drop down naturally and evenly, freeing up the neck. The arms should hang loosely, and there should be no tension in the hands and wrists. All arm movements begin in the muscles located in the middle of the back, not in the shoulders. If, during any of the exercises, you feel tension returning to the neck or shoulders, circle the shoulders a few times in each direction to loosen them up again.

Back and stomach

'Navel to spine' is the Pilates mantra. It is the first step in almost every Pilates exercise for the simple reason that it is the basis of good posture. Stand sideways to the mirror. Does your lower back curve in? Or does your stomach or bottom stick out? Now, try pulling the navel to the spine and watch the change. You should feel lengthened and gently held in. When you exercise in this position, you safeguard your back and strengthen your abdominal muscles.

Buttocks

As you pull the navel to the spine, you will feel your pelvis tilt very slightly upwards. You need to hold this position by gently squeezing the middle muscles in the buttocks. This is the third element in the Pilates 'girdle of strength' or 'central girdle' – the others are the abdominal muscles and the Latissimus dorsi muscles (lats) in the middle of the back. Together, they hold the body in perfect alignment.

Legs and feet

Without pushing your knees too far back, your legs should be straight and elongated. If an exercise calls for a stretched leg, you should feel the stretch all the way up and through to the buttock muscles. There are two basic foot positions for all these exercises. In the first, a flexed foot forms a right angle with the leg. Don't force your toes back, as this can cause cramp, instead, keep them in line with the rest of the foot. In the second position, the foot is pointed. Here the foot stretches away from the ankle in a long, straight line.

Self-assessment: the spine

THE ROLL DOWN (PLACING THE SPINE)

Pilates has often – and rightly – been called 'thinking exercise' for the simple reason that it is a measured, profound technique that calls for a constant awareness of each and every part of your body. In other techniques, a simple side stretch, for instance, may be just that. However, in Pilates, the whole of the body is working. Before you make that stretch you check that the effort of the movement is consolidated by the strength of the central girdle; that there is no tension in the neck or shoulders; and that the movement originates in the correct muscles. Because posture and alignment are central to Pilates, one of the most useful exercises you can do, both to check and correct them, is the Roll Down. It will also show you how tight your hamstring muscles are.

↻ Position two
Gently drop your chin on to your chest, feeling the stretch all the way through your neck and upper back. Let the curve continue, gradually, so that your shoulders and upper back begin to roll forwards.

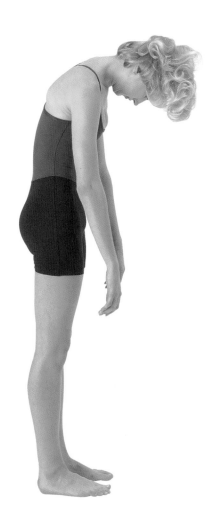

⮌ Position one
Stand sideways on to a mirror with your feet hip-width apart. Check your posture, running through all the points on the previous pages. Your shoulders should be relaxed, dropped down into the back, with your arms hanging comfortably at your sides. Pull the navel to the spine, lift your head so your back is relaxed and lengthened, and check there is no arching in the small of the back.

↻ Position three

Let the curve deepen so it reaches your lower back. Let your arms drop naturally in front of you. Now, without pushing your buttocks back – your legs should be straight and not leaning backwards – let the whole of your upper body hang upside down for a second or two. Try to feel the spaces between the vertebrae as you drop further but don't strain to touch the floor if this does not happen naturally. The weight of your head will automatically stretch out the spine. It may be necessary to bend your knees a little to come back up to standing.

↻ Position four

Come back as slowly as possible, keeping a stretched-out feeling in your back. First, feel the buttock muscles pulling under to place the pelvis and anchor the base of the spine. Now, unroll the spine, vertebra by vertebra, keeping a tall, lengthened position, and drawing the navel to the spine. As your back unrolls, feel your shoulders drop down naturally and, last of all, place your neck and head in line with the spine. You should now be standing in a good posture, stretched and supported by the muscles of the girdle of strength. You can do the Roll Down at the beginning of your exercise session at any level, just to check your posture, or if you feel at any time that you are tense or somehow out of alignment.

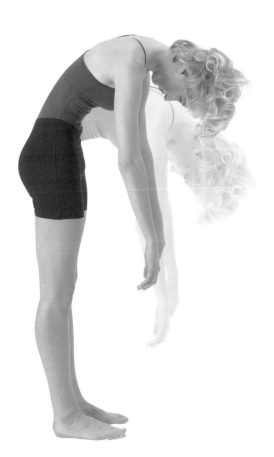

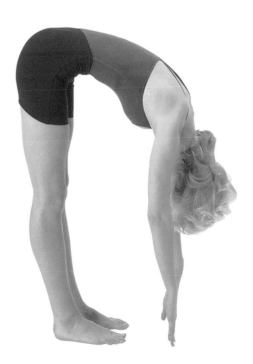

Self-assessment: the upper body

The upper body often seems to attract the stresses of everyday living. Tension can be visible and lead to problems – rigid, bunched muscles, hunched shoulders, a distorted spine, poor breathing and headaches. Pilates technique aims to free this area, giving an elongated spine, relaxed shoulders, a long neck and a gracefully held head.

Start by standing facing the mirror. Is your head lifted up by a long neck, or does it seem to be pushing down into your shoulders? Are your shoulders even, or is one higher? Do they roll forwards making your breastbone sink inwards?

Now stand sideways and look at your reflection. Do the shoulder blades bulge out? Is your head dropping too far forwards or your chin jutting up? You should be able to trace a straight line from your ear through the shoulder down to the hips, if you are standing well.

Try to put yourself in the correct posture using the pictures on pp. 20–21, or use the Roll Down on the previous pages to help you. These two exercises will help you assess any tension and begin to free it up and improve your posture.

SHOULDER LIFT

This simple exercise will be developed later in the book. Here, use it to let the shoulders relax and drop down into their true position. Face a mirror to do this exercise. You should see a gradual change in your shoulder placement by the end of three repetitions.

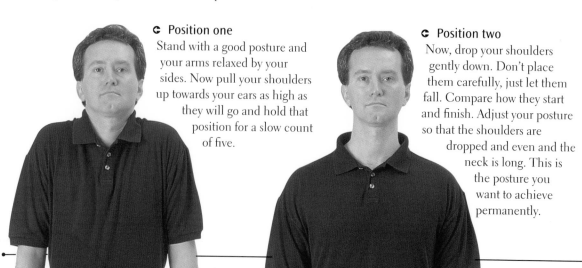

☾ Position one
Stand with a good posture and your arms relaxed by your sides. Now pull your shoulders up towards your ears as high as they will go and hold that position for a slow count of five.

☾ Position two
Now, drop your shoulders gently down. Don't place them carefully, just let them fall. Compare how they start and finish. Adjust your posture so that the shoulders are dropped and even and the neck is long. This is the posture you want to achieve permanently.

ARM PRESSES

This exercise demonstrates where all arm movements should originate. Tension in the neck and shoulders is usually caused by using the wrong muscles to move the arms. Most people, if they lift or stretch their arms in any direction, start by moving their shoulders. In fact, arm movements should come from much lower down in the back, using the lats and lower trapezius, the muscles of the shoulder blades. This will improve posture, reduce tension and make arm movements much more graceful.

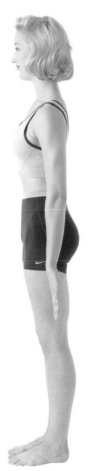

↻ Position one

Stand in front of a mirror with your shoulders and arms relaxed and your head held on a long neck. You are going to move your arms backwards but, before your arms do anything at all, feel the muscles below the shoulder blades (the lats) engage and pull down. You will see your shoulders drop very slightly.

↪ Position two

With your arms straight and your palms facing behind you, move your arms backwards in one motion, palms uppermost. You will feel the lats working. Stretch back, lifting the palms up, very slowly. If your shoulders start to move up or your hands turn in, you have gone too far. If you are doing it correctly, you will feel the chest open at the same time.

Return to the starting position and repeat three to five times. Having located this feeling, always try to use the lats in this way.

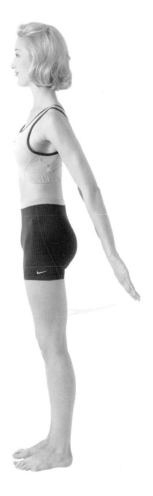

Self-assessment: the central girdle

According to Joseph Pilates, a central core of strength was the essential foundation of all exercise. He called this the 'girdle of strength'. It includes the Latissimus dorsi (lats), as we have seen on the previous pages, the abdomen (the rectus, the external and the internal oblique, and the transversus muscles), the pelvic floor and the buttocks (or gluteus maximus). This is why, in virtually every exercise in this book, before there is any other movement the first instruction is: 'Take a deep breath in and, as you breathe out, draw the navel to the spine.' As the muscles of this central girdle grow stronger, you are able to advance through the Pilates programme in the book. Without this central core of strength, many of the later exercises would be either impossible to complete or would put a strain on the body that could create problems later – most notably in the back.

It is important to notice here that the effort of the exercises is always on the out-breath. In some exercise techniques, including Pilates when taught badly, the effort is put on the in-breath. This causes tension and bunched muscles. By always moving on the out-breath, though, you will achieve the much-desired strong but elongated body without bulging muscles.

The abdominal muscles are often weak and under-used and this can put undue strain on the back. In this technique, the abdominals are strengthened so that they are always held, not just during exercise, but throughout the day – which gives you a much more pleasing shape, as well as a stronger one. The pelvic tilt shown on p. 28 helps you to locate the abdominal muscles and use them correctly. It may seem as if very little is happening but, unless you learn to use these muscles properly, you will not be able to do the more difficult pelvic tilts later on. The surest sign of weak abdominal muscles is that they begin to bulge out with the effort. If they do this, stop immediately.

The first exercise here, the Cossack, uses the Latissimus dorsi (lats) together with the abdominals. It will help you to assess their strength as well as the flexibility of the spine.

THE COSSACK

This exercise appears in chapter four, level one. Here it is used to check on strength and flexibility. You will need to sit or stand in front of a mirror so that you can see exactly what your body is doing. Repeat it two or three times, trying to go a little further each time.

↻ Position one

Sit or stand in front of a mirror and fold your arms loosely so they are parallel with the breastbone. Don't grip hard with your hands as this will create tension in your neck and shoulders, which should feel relaxed and free. Your hips should be facing forwards – they do not move throughout the exercise. Breathe in and, as you breathe out, draw the lats down into the back and draw the navel to the spine.

☉ Position two

Keeping your hips facing the mirror, turn slowly from the waist, feeling as if your body is rotating around a straight spine. Let the turn move into the upper back and, finally, the head. Don't let your shoulders tense up.

☉ Position three

As you breathe in, come back to the starting point. Check your shoulders – they should be level and relaxed.

☉ Position four

Repeat, turning slowly to the other side. Return to the centre and repeat two or three times to each side, checking your shoulders each time you reach the central position.

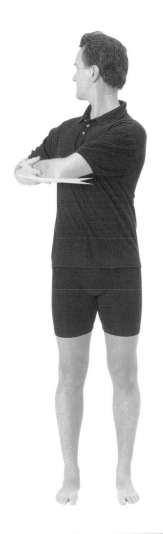
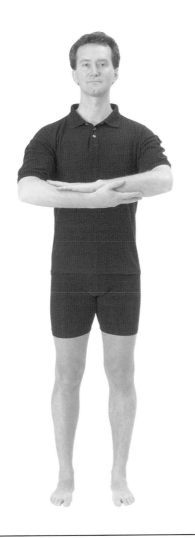
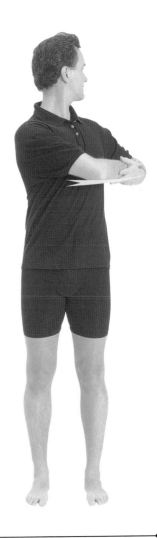

PELVIC TILT

This is the same as the very first of the pelvic tilt exercises that you do in chapter four, level one. Here it is used to help you assess your posture and to locate the abdominals. Begin by lying flat on the floor, with your legs bent at the knees and your feet about 7cm (3in) apart. Your arms should be relaxed at your sides, with no tension in the shoulders or neck. Check how much space there is between the small of your back and the floor. Ideally, it should be only a small hollow. Now, breathe in and, as you breathe out, draw the navel to the spine – you will feel the hollow reducing. It is this feeling that you want to recreate in the exercises throughout the book.

↺ Position one

Lie with your feet up on a chair so that your knees form a right angle. The hollow in your back will be smaller than when your legs are on the floor – your aim in this position is to have a flat but soft back. Place a rolled-up towel or cushion between your thighs – this helps keep the pelvis centred throughout the exercise.

↻ Position two

Take a deep breath and, as you breathe out, draw the navel to the spine, feeling your back drop down towards the floor. As you do this, gently curl the base of the spine away from the floor – this will help you to feel a 'scoop' in the abdomen. You will need this motion later when you do further pelvic tilts where you curl up off the floor.

SELF-HELP QUESTIONNAIRE

Going through this chapter, you may have noticed that some areas of your posture need working on. Don't be dismayed; after all, if your posture was perfect, you wouldn't need help. Ask yourself if you can identify any of the following common problems, and when you are able, use the suggested exercises from chapter four to remedy them. Always do the warm-up first.

1 When you stand sideways to the mirror, does your:
⮑ Stomach protrude?
⮑ Bottom stick out?
⮑ Lower back curve inwards?
⮑ Chin jut out and tilt upwards?

If so, you need to work on the girdle of strength and firm up the abdominals, buttock muscles, hamstrings and lats. Use the exercises on pp. 64, 68–69, 91, 92–93, 96–97, 100, 108, 109 and 133.

2 Are your shoulders stiff with tension?
⮑ Do they roll forwards, giving you round shoulders?
⮑ Are they pulled tightly back. giving you a stiff back and neck?

If so, you need shoulder exercises. See pp. 52–53, 60–61, 63 and 80.

3 Are your legs straight and do they feel elongated?
If not, use the exercises for toning the legs on pp. 70–71, 88–91 and 116–117.

4 Do the muscles above your knees droop down?
If so, practise the remedial legs exercises on pp. 72–73, 98–99 and 129.

5 When you did the Roll Down on p. 22, did your lower back and hamstrings feel tight?
If so, stretch them out with the exercises on pp. 52, 100 and 133.

6 Were you able to do the pelvic tilts on p. 28 without your abdominals popping out?
If not, use the exercises from the warm-up on pp. 48–49.

7 Did you remember to breathe throughout the self-assessment exercises?
If not, practise the warm-up scarf exercise on p. 50.

Remember that **STRAIN AND PAIN ARE NOT THE AIM**. Just do what you can and you will notice a gradual but perceptible postural improvement.

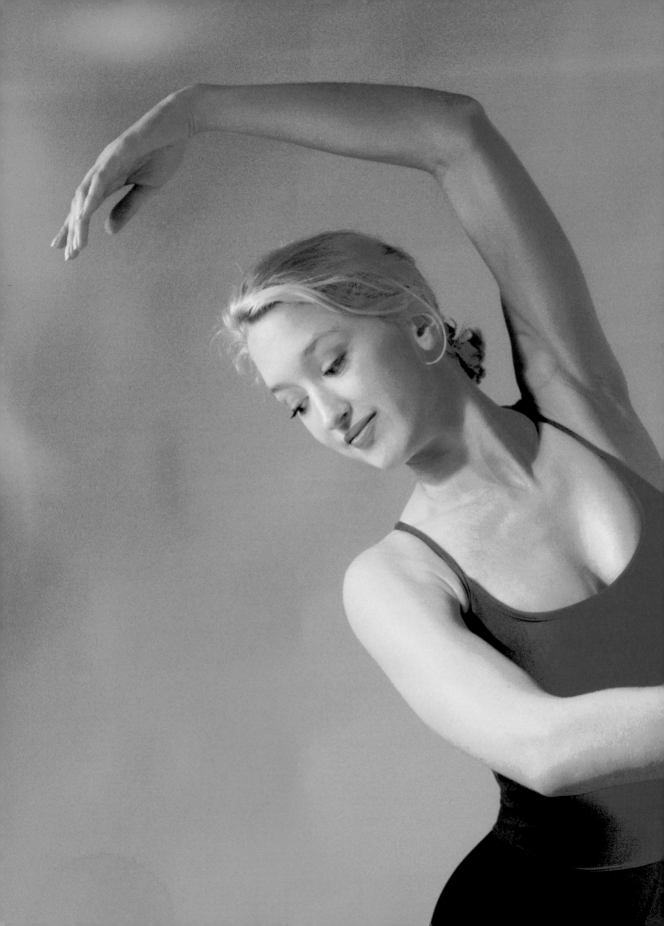

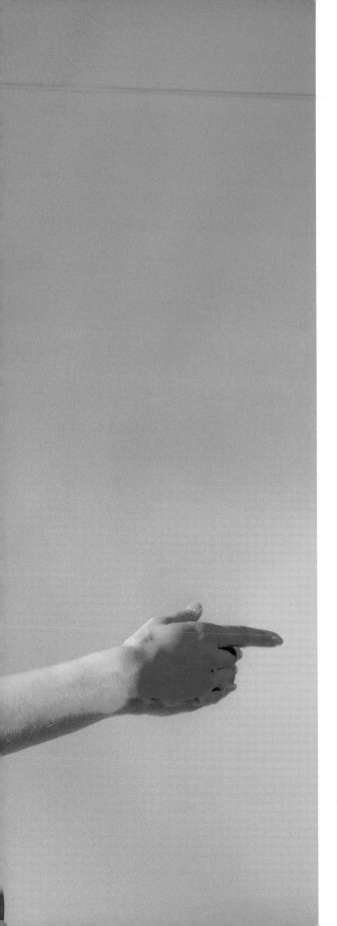

Chapter Three

The Pilates Studio

• •

A Pilates studio is unlike any other gym. The atmosphere is calm and quiet and the music classical and soothing; light years away from the pumping rhythms of the aerobics studio.

Here, the benefits of the lengthening and strengthening exercises of the Pilates technique are achieved more quickly by working against the resistance of springs, pulleys and weights. Under the guidance of an experienced Pilates teacher, posture can be realigned perfectly while the whole body is toned and firmed. Problem areas such as flabby arms or stiff hip joints can be addressed safely, and tensions of both mind and body float gently away.

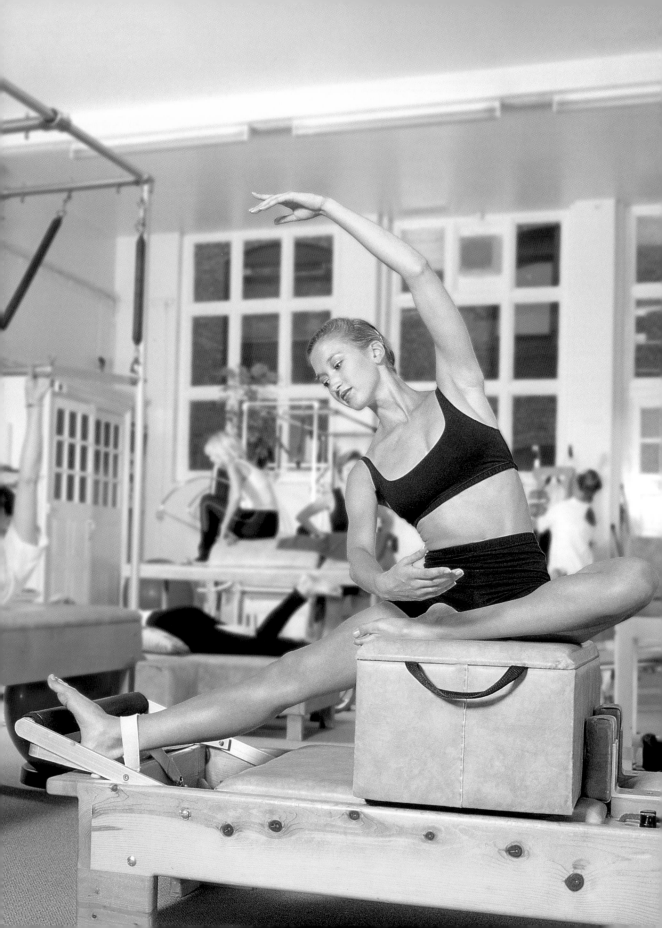

Everyone has a different body shape with particular capabilities, bad habits and ultimate potential. So, in the Pilates studio, everyone works according to a programme individually designed to suit their own body. While people can have unrealistic expectations of any exercise system, it is certainly true that Pilates can radically alter your body shape, within your particular anatomical limits.

There are two great advantages of going to a Pilates studio even if most of your exercising takes place at home. Firstly, when working against the resistance of the machines you often become more aware of what a particular exercise is expecting of your body. On the plié machine, for instance, you will probably be aware of the muscles of your thighs and buttocks working more intensely than when you do pliés at home, perhaps at a deeper level within the muscle or through a greater stretch. Once you have recognised this feeling, you can incorporate the same level of intensity into your own programme at home.

Secondly, and perhaps even more importantly, you get the individual attention of a teacher who will watch you throughout, making adjustments to your posture, demonstrating breathing and the correct movements, and giving you new exercises as you become stronger and more supple. This means you are learning the exercise properly, thus giving you more confidence when using it on your own at home.

EXERCISING ON PILATES EQUIPMENT

The lion's share of this book, chapter four, shows you how to exercise the Pilates way at home. In this chapter, you can see how those exercises relate to the Pilates studio and what you can expect to do when you go there. All the studio photographs shown here were taken at Alan Herdman's studio in London; and they use only around half of the available equipment. If at all possible, try to go to just a few classes with a qualified instructor. Even if there is no local, fully-equipped Pilates studio, there are now many 'matwork' classes where Pilates technique is taught without equipment.

SIDE STRETCH

This is a marvellous stretch for all of the muscles along your side from the hip to the ribcage. In the studio (opposite) it is performed sitting on a box on top of the plié machine. See pp. 42–43 for full, step-by-step instructions.

At home you can adapt it using a chair. The home exercise is shown in full on p. 56, and is part of the warm-up that you use to begin every exercise session.

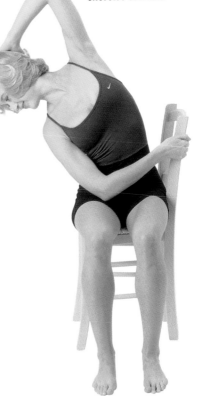

The girdle of strength

The Pilates 'girdle of strength' is centred on the abdominal muscles and extends out to the buttocks and the lats, or Latissimus dorsi, the muscles in the back that control shoulder and arm movements. The words 'breathe out, draw the navel to the spine' are repeated like a mantra in the Pilates studio, at the start of nearly every exercise. The reason for this is that the strength needed for the exercises originates in the abdominal muscles. If these muscles are not in control of a movement, then other muscles such as those in the back, neck or shoulders attempt to carry the burden and can be damaged. However, by using the abdominals correctly, and only as far as they are able to go at the time, you will develop strength and postural awareness. The abdominal curls (or Roll) Down in this chapter show how the muscles are strengthened and stretched in the Pilates studio.

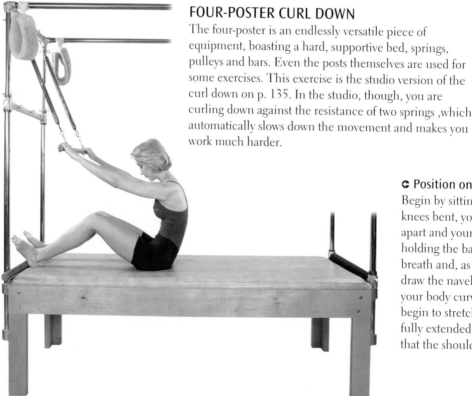

FOUR-POSTER CURL DOWN
The four-poster is an endlessly versatile piece of equipment, boasting a hard, supportive bed, springs, pulleys and bars. Even the posts themselves are used for some exercises. This exercise is the studio version of the curl down on p. 135. In the studio, though, you are curling down against the resistance of two springs ,which automatically slows down the movement and makes you work much harder.

↺ Position one
Begin by sitting up with your knees bent, your feet a hip-width apart and your hands loosely holding the bar. Take a deep breath and, as you breathe out, draw the navel to the spine, letting your body curve. Your arms will begin to stretch. When they are fully extended, engage the lats so that the shoulders pull down.

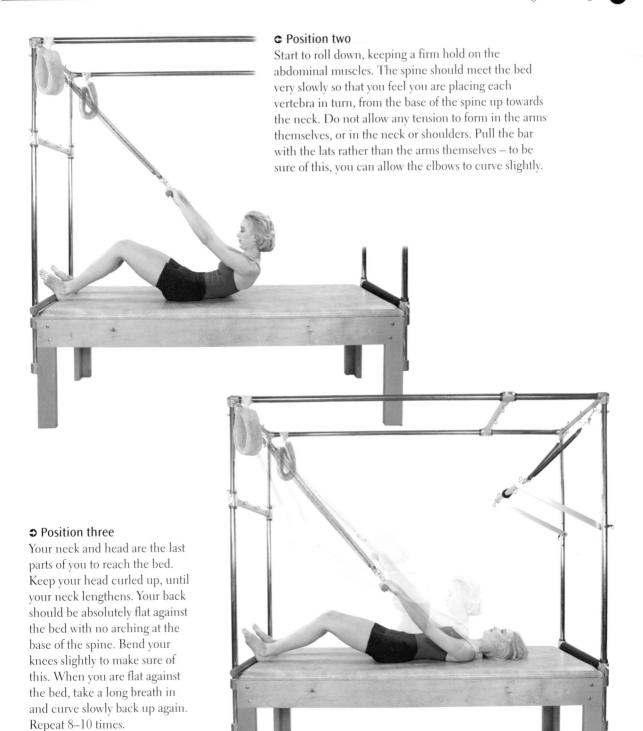

⟲ Position two

Start to roll down, keeping a firm hold on the abdominal muscles. The spine should meet the bed very slowly so that you feel you are placing each vertebra in turn, from the base of the spine up towards the neck. Do not allow any tension to form in the arms themselves, or in the neck or shoulders. Pull the bar with the lats rather than the arms themselves – to be sure of this, you can allow the elbows to curve slightly.

⟳ Position three

Your neck and head are the last parts of you to reach the bed. Keep your head curled up, until your neck lengthens. Your back should be absolutely flat against the bed with no arching at the base of the spine. Bend your knees slightly to make sure of this. When you are flat against the bed, take a long breath in and curve slowly back up again. Repeat 8–10 times.

ABDOMINAL CURLS ON A BOX

This is a much more advanced abdominals exercise.
It takes place on the plié machine, which has a box
placed on top of it to form a seat, while the feet are
tucked under a strap. In this exercise, you do not work
against the resistance of springs, but you do hold a pole
which keeps the arms stretched and level throughout.
This is a very tough exercise and one that requires real
strength in the abdominal muscles and a good deal of
postural awareness.

⮑ Position one

Begin by sitting on the box, with your legs straight and
the feet sufficiently flexed to keep the strap in place.
Sit very tall on the box, pulling up out of your hips so
that the buttocks and legs are working. Making sure
that your back stays absolutely straight, with your neck
in line with your spine, raise your arms, bringing
the pole above your head. There should be
no tension in the shoulders or neck; you
should be able to turn your head freely
from side to side. Take a deep breath in.

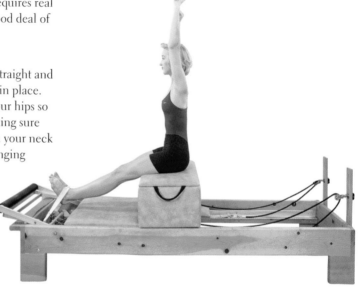

⮑ Position two

As you breathe out, draw the navel to the spine
and start to curl your back down so that the
abdominal muscles scoop, and your head and
shoulders curve gently towards your body.
At the same time, lower your arms gradually
until they are stretched out in front of you.

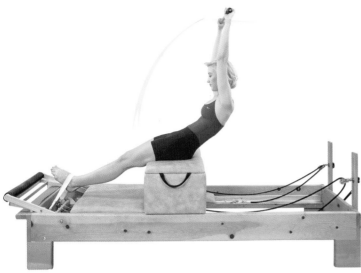

↻ Position three

Holding the curve – don't let the abdominal muscles pop out during the next movement – raise the pole above your head until your arms are stretched up towards the ceiling again. Don't let any tension form in your neck or shoulders, or let the effort go into the small of your back.

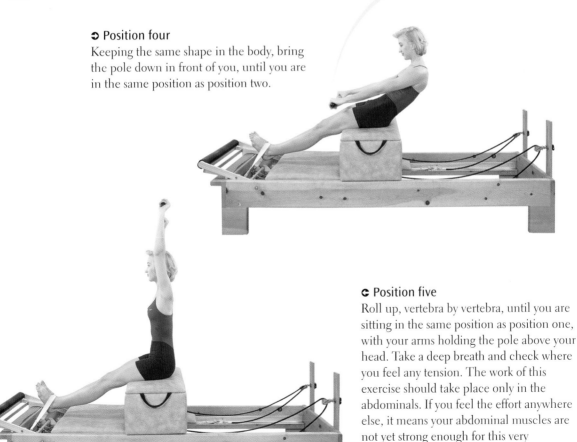

➲ Position four

Keeping the same shape in the body, bring the pole down in front of you, until you are in the same position as position two.

↻ Position five

Roll up, vertebra by vertebra, until you are sitting in the same position as position one, with your arms holding the pole above your head. Take a deep breath and check where you feel any tension. The work of this exercise should take place only in the abdominals. If you feel the effort anywhere else, it means your abdominal muscles are not yet strong enough for this very strenuous exercise. Repeat 8–10 times.

The lats and torso

The 'lats' or Latissimus dorsi, are the uppermost section of the Pilates 'girdle of strength' – and are frequently forgotten by most of us. The lats are the muscles behind the shoulder blades, and should form the source of all arm and shoulder movement. Most people use the shoulders themselves instead of the lats when they move their arms. This results in tension in the neck and shoulders, often with accompanying tension headaches. Together with strong abdominal muscles, proper use of the lats virtually guarantees good posture. They are muscles that are definitely worth remembering and bringing back into use.

The exercises shown here engage the lats and the trapezius muscles above them, and stretch out the upper torso. This stretching inevitably brings a great feeling of release and freedom in the upper body, especially to those of us who sit with hunched posture and rounded shoulders.

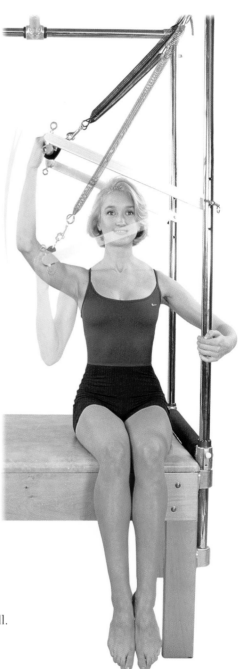

LOCATING THE LATS

This is a good exercise for locating the lats and learning how to use them properly. It relates to the one on p. 62. Ideally, you should do them both in front of a mirror – this enables you to see what your shoulders are doing. If you're exercising properly, they should be doing nothing. The work takes place in the back so, as the bar raises and lowers, you shouldn't be able to see any movement at all in the shoulder itself.

Position one

Sit squarely, with your knees together, your shoulders dropped down into the back and your spine straight. Breathe in and, as you breathe out, draw the navel towards the spine. Holding the bar lightly with the fingertips, lower it by drawing down the lats.

Position two

Allow the bar to return to the starting position. Feel the movement in the lats only, and keep the shoulders quite still. Repeat 8–10 times.

Stretching out the upper torso

This is the studio version of the exercise on pp. 122–123. Try to stretch the upper body without tensing the shoulders and, in position two, keep your arms touching the bed for as long as you can, to release the shoulder joint and free up the back. The sensation of the stretch is wonderfully elongating.

Position one

Lie on your back with the knees raised, the feet flat, and the whole length of the spine pressed into the bed. Stretch out your arms to hold the bar, without tension. Breathe in and, as you breathe out, pull the navel further into the bed and start to draw the bar down towards you.

Position two

As your upper arms reach the bed, start to circle your elbows out so that the bar goes further away from your body. Keep your upper arms in contact with the bed for as long as possible. When your arms cannot stay on the bed any longer, breathe out and stretch them out behind your head, still keeping your spine flat on the bed. Breathe in, and return to position two. Breathe out, and return to the starting position. Repeat 8–10 times.

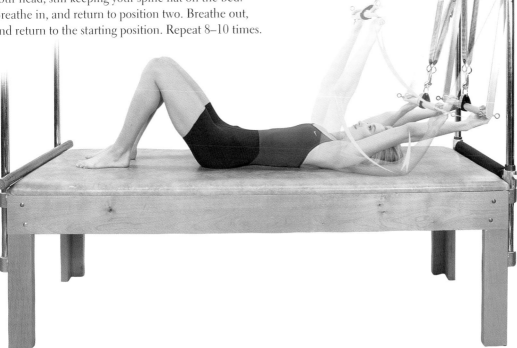

The arms and upper body

These exercises are all slow, small and deceptively simple. The upper torso exercises use the lats and the trapezius muscles while opening up and releasing the chest. The arm exercises are very similar to those on pp. 74–75 but, as the body is raised off the ground on a piece of equipment called the barrel, it gives the arms a greater stretch.

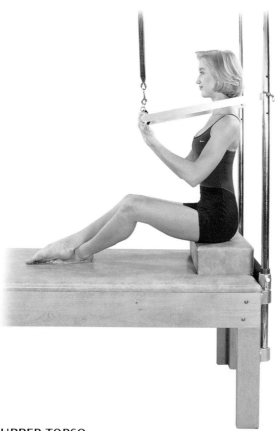 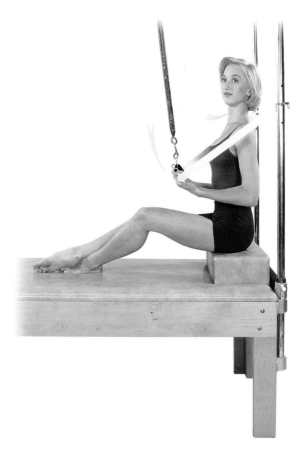

UPPER TORSO

⌂ Position one
Sitting very tall on a small box, with your legs stretched out and crossed at the ankles, place your fingertips loosely on the bar. Your head should be in line with a long straight spine and there should be no tension anywhere in the body.

⌂ Position two
Breathe in and, as you breathe out, draw the bar down very slowly, feeling your chest open, your neck lengthen and your head lift and turn towards your left shoulder. Return to the centre and alternate right and left.

TRICEPS EXERCISE

The triceps are the muscles in the back of your upper arms, and this exercise is a boon for flabby upper arms.

↻ Position one

Lie with your knees bent and your back flat against the barrel. Check there is no arch in the small of your back. Hold the weight in both hands so that it drops down towards your chest.

↻ Position two

Breathe in and, as you breathe out, draw the navel to the spine and, in one smooth movement, lift the weight over your head as far as you can. Breathe in and return to the starting position.

ARM OPENINGS

Here, you use two weights of up to 1kg each. This exercise not only tones the arm muscles, but also opens up the back and chest and releases the shoulder joints.

↪ Position one

Lie on the barrel with your knees raised, the whole of your spine flat against the barrel, and your arms in a wide curve with your hands meeting above the chest. Feel as if you are holding a beach ball within the curve of your arms.

↪ Position two

Breathe in and, as you breathe out, draw the navel to the spine and open your arms outwards, still retaining the curve. Breathe in and return to the starting position.

USING ARM WEIGHTS

These exercises relate directly to those in chapter four. All the arm exercises given up to then start off without weights, because you only add them when you have built up some strength. You can substitute cans of beans for the weights, but working against any form of weight is beneficial, especially as we age. Weight work can actually prevent osteoporosis in menopausal and post-menopausal women. Use weights of up to 1kg.

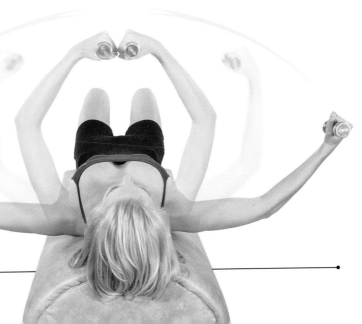

SIDE STRETCHES

This advanced exercise requires a great deal of strength and postural awareness. It stretches out both sides of the body in turn and has a very graceful, dancer-like feeling to it. Again, it uses a box on the plié machine and the position is secured by the foot strap.

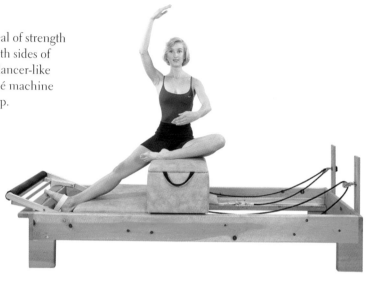

➲ Position one

Sit on the box with your right foot tucked under the strap and your left leg bent and resting on the box. Your back should be completely straight, with your head lifted and in line with your spine. The right arm is raised in a graceful curve, and the left arm is curved in front of the body.

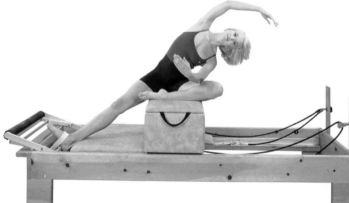

↻ Position two

Take a deep breath in and, as you breathe out, draw the navel to the spine and bend smoothly over to the left. Your arms and legs should remain in exactly the same relationship to the body as in position one.

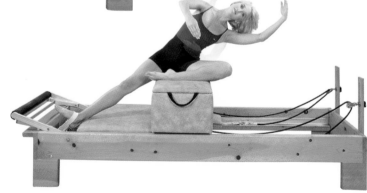

➲ Position three

Now reverse the arms so that the left is extended in a curve away from your body and the right is curved in front.

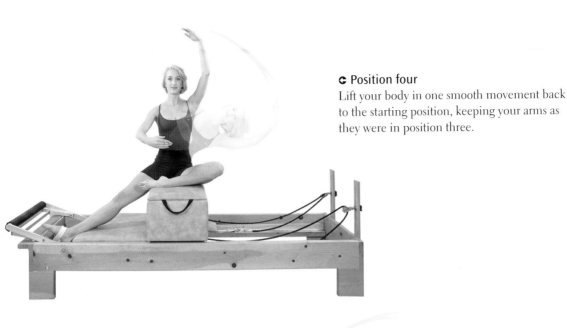

↻ Position four
Lift your body in one smooth movement back to the starting position, keeping your arms as they were in position three.

↺ Position five
Take another breath and, as you breathe out, bend the other way so that your left arm is curving down towards your right foot. Keep drawing the navel to the spine.

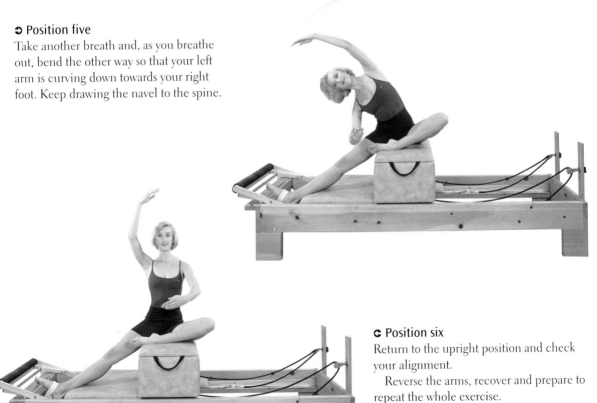

↻ Position six
Return to the upright position and check your alignment.

Reverse the arms, recover and prepare to repeat the whole exercise.

Pliés

Pliés are one of the fundamental ballet exercises. Though they may look like simple knee bends, they are actually much more complex than this. When performed correctly, the plié uses most of the body. Because they are complex movements, they are not brought into the home routine until level three (pp. 130–131), by which time you will have greater body awareness and will be able to focus on several areas at the same time. In the studio, you do them on the plié machine which helps in various ways. Firstly, because you are lying down, your spine is straight and you are less prone to bad posture and injury. Secondly, working against springs is harder and enables you to become aware of the muscles in the abdominals, legs and buttocks that you should be using. As you can add up to four springs for resistance, the work is more intense and your muscles become toned up faster.

PLIÉS: FIRST POSITION
↻ Position one
Begin with the bed of the plié machine close to the foot rest. Place your feet so that your toes are on the foot rest and your heels are together, forming a V-shape. This position for the feet is called 'turned out' and this means that your whole leg follows the same direction. Without exaggerating the position, your knees should be facing slightly outwards and your legs should feel the turn-out all the way from the hip socket downwards. Make sure your back and neck are in a long straight line, and your arms and shoulders are relaxed at your sides.

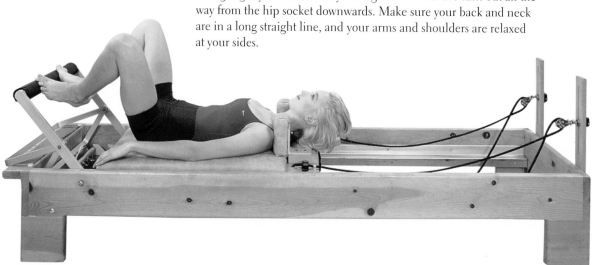

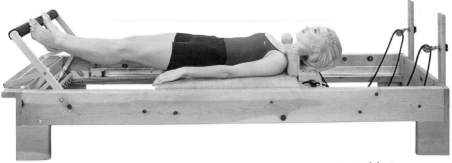

☊ Position two

Breathe in, then breathe out, draw the navel to the spine and push away from the foot rest until your legs are straight. As you push, feel the turn-out strongly in your thighs and buttocks. The muscles should feel as if they are wrapping around your leg – imagine the inner thigh trying to face uppermost. Breathe in and return to position one.

PLIÉS: SECOND POSITION

➲ Position one

This time, position your feet so that your heels are on the outside edges of the foot rest. With your knees dropping out to the sides, you should feel a sense of openness in the hip socket. Check your spinal alignment before you move on to the next stage.

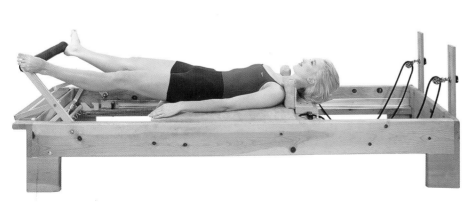

↺ Position two

Breathe in and, as you breathe out, draw the navel to the spine and push away from the foot rest until your legs are straight. Feel the turn-out. Breathe in to return to position one. Aim to repeat each position 10 times.

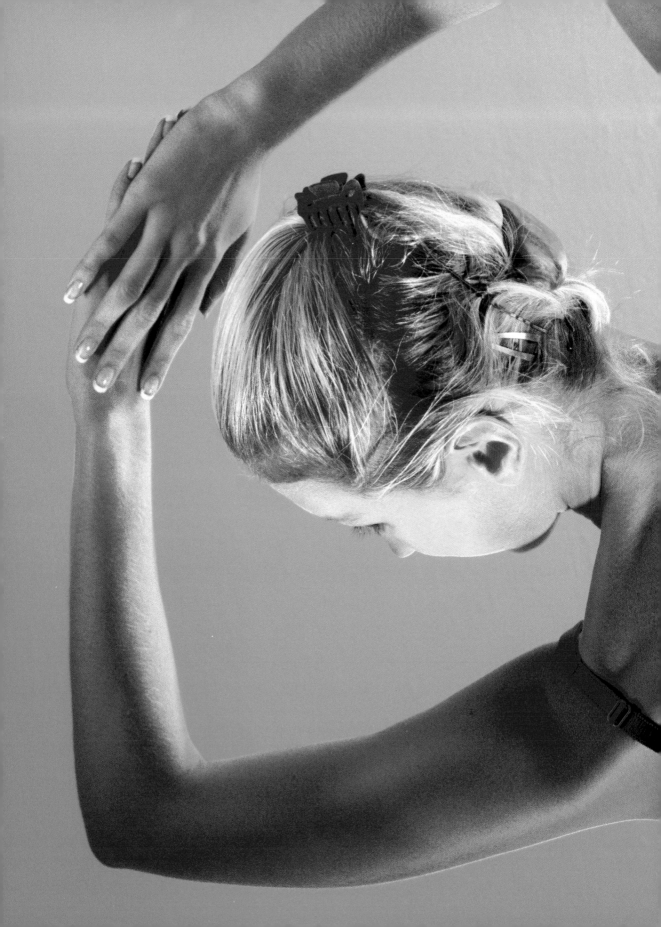

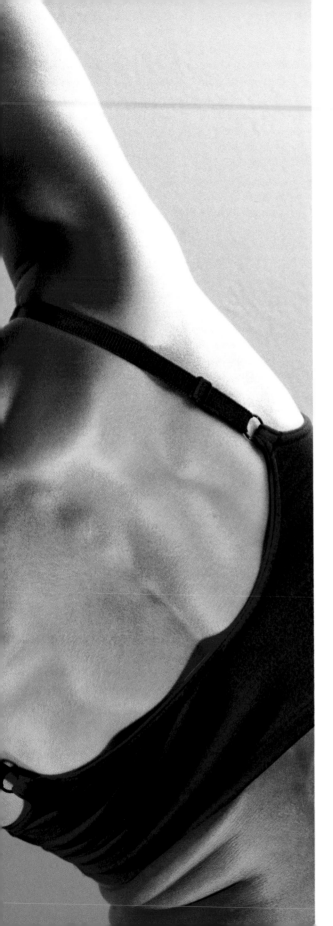

Chapter Four

The Pilates Workout

This workout is the safest, most thorough way to achieve the shape you've always wanted. You will look and feel better within weeks and, on completion, have a dancer's strong, lean, flexible physique.

The programme's golden rule is: don't rush it. Always warm up before you exercise – this trains your body's memory to use the correct muscles every time. Don't be tempted to advance to another level until you have truly mastered the current one – you may strain your muscles and joints. Each level is designed to strengthen your body as an integrated whole. Aim to exercise three times a week in a tranquil environment. Feel your body changing – and enjoy it.

The warm-up session

The Pilates warm-up is quite different from other warm-ups. **Because Pilates exercises are so precise, it is vital to ensure you are moving correctly, and the warm-up helps you to locate, isolate and develop all of the key areas to be used in the exercises to come.** The same warm-up applies to all three levels, because all three use the same muscles, though with varying degrees of difficulty and complexity. However, there is another good reason for the warm-up repetition.

As every dancer knows, the body, not just the mind, has a memory, and by repeating these movements regularly, they will inform not only your exercise session but every single movement of your daily life.

YOU WILL NEED

Essentials
- *Comfortable clothing.*
- *A soft carpet, towel or yoga mat to lie on.*
- *A long scarf.*
- *A medium-sized towel.*
- *Firm cushions of various sizes.*
- *A chair or stool (your knees must bend at 90° when seated on it).*
- *An item of household furniture that supports your weight, e.g. a table or door frame.*

Extras
- *Hand-held weights, either 1kg (2lb) dumb-bells or ordinary food cans.*
- *Strap-on 1kg leg weights.*
- *A lightweight pole or broom handle.*
- *Stability ball.*

BREATHING

Though the following exercise may suggest that little is happening, it is fundamental. Because deep rhythmic breathing is so important, and indeed shapes all of the exercises, it is vital to start by establishing proper breathing. You may find slow classical music will help keep your breathing steady and rhythmic. Or, if you prefer, set the pace by your own breathing.

↻ Position one

Lie on your back with your feet up on a chair, and your knees forming a right angle. Make sure you lie straight, with no tension in your neck and shoulders. Place a rolled-up towel or cushion between your knees. Make a diamond shape with your hands over the abdominal muscles, and rest your head on a book.

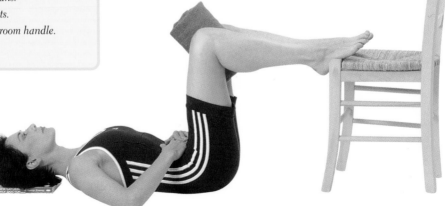

⟳ Position two

Now breathe very slowly and deeply, feeling each breath reach the lungs so that your ribs and back widen with the inwards breath. Try to create a constant, slow, deep rhythm. This is how you need to breathe throughout the exercises. Repeat for 10 slow, deep breaths.

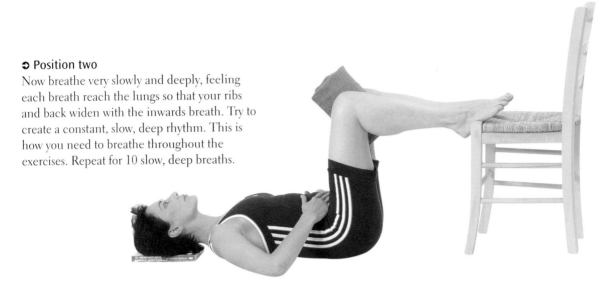

THE SCOOP

This is a continuation of the previous exercise and transforms the breathing into a movement.

↻ Lie on the floor with your spine lengthened, the small of the back touching the floor and your neck and shoulders relaxed. Place a cushion or rolled-up towel between your knees.

Breathe in and, as you breathe out, draw the navel to the spine so that the abdominal muscles are scooped into a spoon shape. Do this 10 times, trying to extend the scoop further each time.

THE SCOOP

The Scoop teaches the basis of all pelvic tilt exercises and you can use it to feel these muscles in their entirety. The more abdominal muscles you can engage the better – these muscles almost reach the pelvic floor area and can be scooped up the whole way.

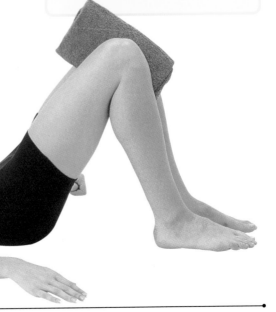

THE SCARF

This is another exercise to help achieve the correct breathing you need for Pilates. Keep the scarf taut – but not tight – throughout, and it will help you focus on your breath.

↪ Position one

Stand, or sit on a chair or stool, so that your knees form a right angle when your feet are flat the floor. Your toes should point straight forwards. Take a scarf and wrap it around your upper body so that it covers the whole depth of your ribs. Cross it in front of you and hold one end in each hand.

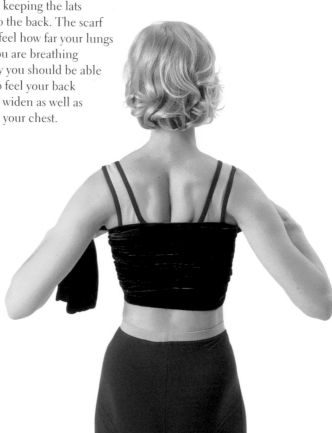

↩ Position two

Take a deep breath in and fill your lungs with air, keeping the lats pulled down into the back. The scarf will help you to feel how far your lungs expand – if you are breathing properly you should be able to feel your back widen as well as your chest.

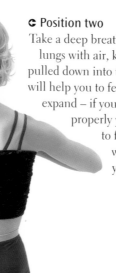

↪ Position three

Breathe out and feel your body empty of air. Keep the scarf taut. Repeat for 10 breaths, trying to expand your lungs a little further each time.

DOMING

Most people hardly use the muscles in their feet, which often results in inflexibility. This exercise shows you how to release 'frozen' feet – keep the image of a cat drawing in its claws in your mind and you'll have the right idea. It is also a good exercise for getting your foot working properly again if you have had an injury. You should do it with bare feet.

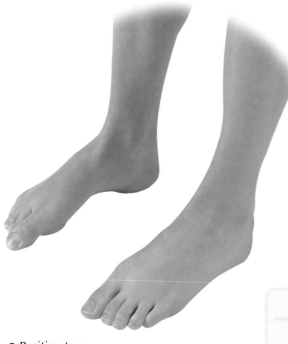

○ Position one
Sit on a chair with your knees bent at right angles and your feet flat on the floor a hips-width apart.

○ Position two
Draw your toes back against the floor so that the instep lifts but the heel stays firmly on the floor. Don't expect a big movement, especially at first. Do not let your toes curl under. Hold the lift for a few seconds before straightening your toes and returning to the starting postion. Repeat 10 times.

FOOT MASSAGE

After doming, you can give yourself a foot massage. This can be very relaxing, especially if you are prone to cramp. Start by gently stroking the whole of your foot. Then apply a firmer pressure by circling your thumbs all over the sole. Finally, apply the same pressure on top of your foot between each of the toes. Pull each toe out from its base, stretching it gently and smoothly.

Releasing the back and neck

The following two exercises release tension stored in the back and the neck. These are problem areas for many people, who can often be unaware that any such tension exists. Once you have freed up the back and the neck, your posture will be improved instantly.

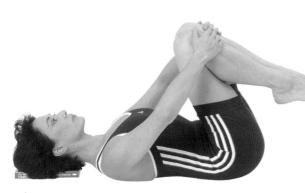

KNEE TO CHEST

You will feel the lower vertebrae open up as you do this exercise.

↻ Position one

Lie on your back so that your whole spine is touching the floor. Bend and lift your knees, keeping them slightly apart, in line with your hips. Draw the navel gently to the spine and hold this position throughout the exercise. Place your hands just below, not on, your knees.

↻ Position three

Breathe in and, as you breathe out, gently draw both knees to your chest, keeping your arms wide. Make sure your entire spine remains on the floor. Feel your back and chest open out as you do this. Repeat in the same sequence – right, then left, then knees together – 10 times.

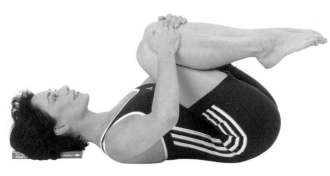

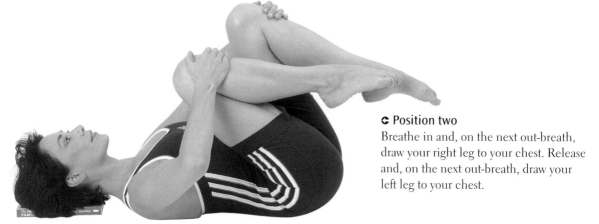

↻ Position two

Breathe in and, on the next out-breath, draw your right leg to your chest. Release and, on the next out-breath, draw your left leg to your chest.

HIP ROLLS – BEGINNERS

This is the first of the hip rolls – you will find later versions throughout the book. In this first stage, concentrate on releasing the lower back and feeling the stretch across the abdomen.

➲ Position one

Lie on your back with your knees bent and pointing to the ceiling and your feet together on the floor. Put your hands on your abdominals to help you feel them stretch. Keep your back and neck long and relaxed.

☾ Position two

Breathe in and, as you breathe out, roll your knees to one side, keeping your buttocks glued to the floor and your knees together. You will not be able to go very far but you should still feel a stretch across the abdominal oblique muscles.

➲ Position three

Breathe in to return to the centre and check your position. Breathe out, and repeat on the other side. Alternate 10 rolls to each side.

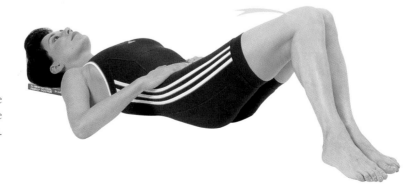

Releasing the upper body

These exercises are very good for anyone who has a tendency to store tension in the shoulders, neck or back. They release the upper body and help to get the lats working properly – the muscles that you should be using to initiate arm movements, rather than the shoulders.

↻ Position two

Now, breathe in and lift up your shoulders towards your ears.

SHOULDER SHRUGS

In this exercise you can lift your shoulders rather than pull them down into the back.

↪ Position one

Sit on a chair in front of a mirror, with your feet flat on the floor and facing forwards. If you have a bolster cushion, stand this on its end between your knees to help stabilise the pelvis. Let your arms hang down relaxed at your sides.

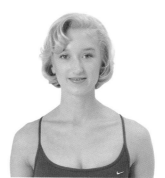
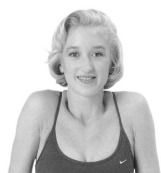

As you draw the arms back, feel the lats pulling down and squeezing together.

↪ Position three

As you breathe out, lower your shoulders and gently stretch your hands down to the floor. Rotate your arms inwards and stretch them behind you – but not too far. If you are doing it properly, this will open up the chest and strengthen the muscles below the shoulder blades. Repeat 10 times.

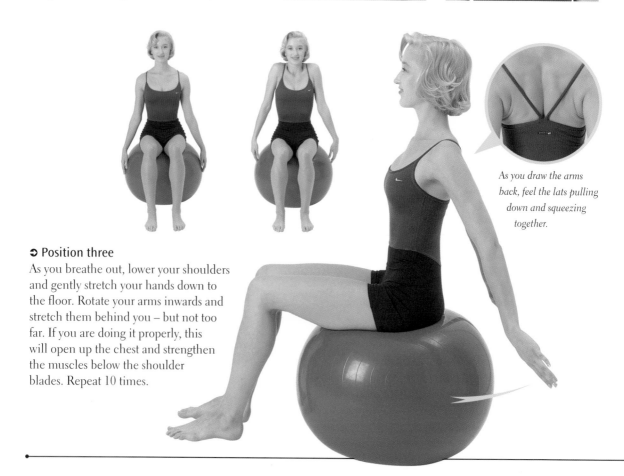

NOSE FIGURE OF EIGHT

The movement involved in this exercise is so small that it looks almost as if nothing is happening, but it actually involves a great deal of concentration. While your mind is involved in controlling the movement, the back of the neck relaxes without your noticing.

↻ Position one

Lie on your back with your knees bent, your back soft and a book beneath your head. Place your arms down by your sides, draw the navel gently towards the spine and squeeze your lower buttock muscles. Hold this position throughout the exercise.

↺ Position two

Focus all of your attention on the tip of your nose and make it trace a figure of eight in the air. Imagine you are drawing on a blackboard. This is only a tiny movement – your face does not turn from side to side. Do 10 figures of eight in one direction, then reverse it and do 10 more. You may find that closing your eyes helps you focus on the movement.

SIDE STRETCHES – BEGINNERS

This is the first of two side-stretching exercises. This one concentrates on the area from the waist to the elbows. The second one, which you perform standing, takes the stretch down through the hips too.

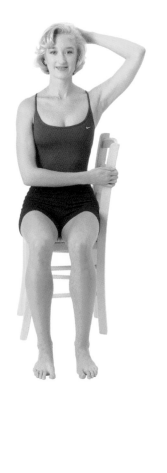

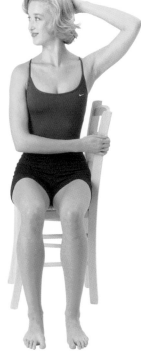

↻ Positions two and three

Take a deep breath in and, as you breathe out, turn your head to the right, away from the chair to avoid tensing your neck. Gently stretch your left side, elbow first, up to the ceiling and then dipping down towards the floor in a big curve. Breathe in to return to the starting position and repeat 10 times on each side.

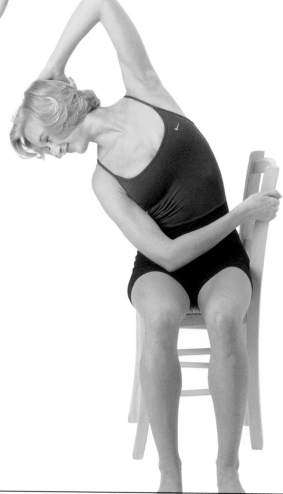

↻ Position one

Sit in a dining chair with your left side against its back. Place your right hand on the chair back so that your arm crosses in front of your body. Put your left hand behind your head. Make sure your body is square and facing forwards, with your knees a hip-width apart and the toes pointing forwards.

SIDE STRETCHES – ELEMENTARY

In this second side stretch, this time in the standing position, you take the stretch further. The greater the distance between you and your support, the further you will be able to stretch.

⟳ Position one

Hold onto a well-anchored chair or a door frame and stand about two feet away from it. Your feet should be apart, your shoulders dropped and you should have no tension in the upper body.

⟲⟳ Position two

Breathe in and, as you breathe out, stretch away from the chair, letting your outer arm describe a wide circle until the hand reaches back over your head. Feel the stretch all the way through your side – keep your head turned towards the chair during this movement to avoid tensing your neck. Return to the starting position and repeat 10 times on each side.

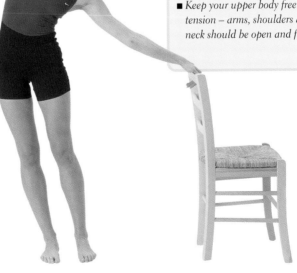

CHECK BOX

- *Keep your feet slightly apart and flat on the floor throughout.*
- *Don't let your body twist – your hips should face squarely to the front throughout.*
- *Keep your upper body free from tension – arms, shoulders and neck should be open and free.*

The Pilates Workout: level one

Words of Wisdom

'Perform your exercises regularly for only three months, and you will find your body development approaching the ideal.'
JOSEPH PILATES

Level one is undoubtedly the most important stage of your Pilates programme. It is here that you learn how to use your body correctly, and the new way of moving that you master is the basis of all the more complex exercises to come.

For this reason alone, don't hurry to move on. By learning to move each part of your body with precision, you will tone and strengthen your muscles as well as improve your posture.

Right from the start, you should establish your exercise routine as a time for quiet concentration. Unplug the telephone or put on the answer machine. Find yourself a warm, comfortable space and put on some quiet, classical music. This will help you to slow down. Above all, remember that these exercises are to be done rhythmically and very slowly.

Your goals for level one

- *Concentrate, first and foremost, on your alignment and posture.*

- *If you feel you are standing or sitting incorrectly or you can feel muscles tensing up, repeat the posture exercises on pp. 20–28 until you feel your placement is as it should be.*

- *Don't rush any of the exercises, even if they feel easy.*

- *Concentrate instead on making each one precise and controlled.*

- *Keep your awareness on your whole body and don't let any one part take over.*

- *Always check that the whole of your body is in the correct position, relaxed and lengthened.*

- *Focus on your breathing – it should be deep, slow and rhythmical, with all the effort performed on the out-breath.*

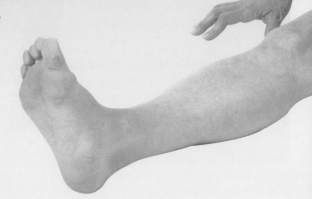

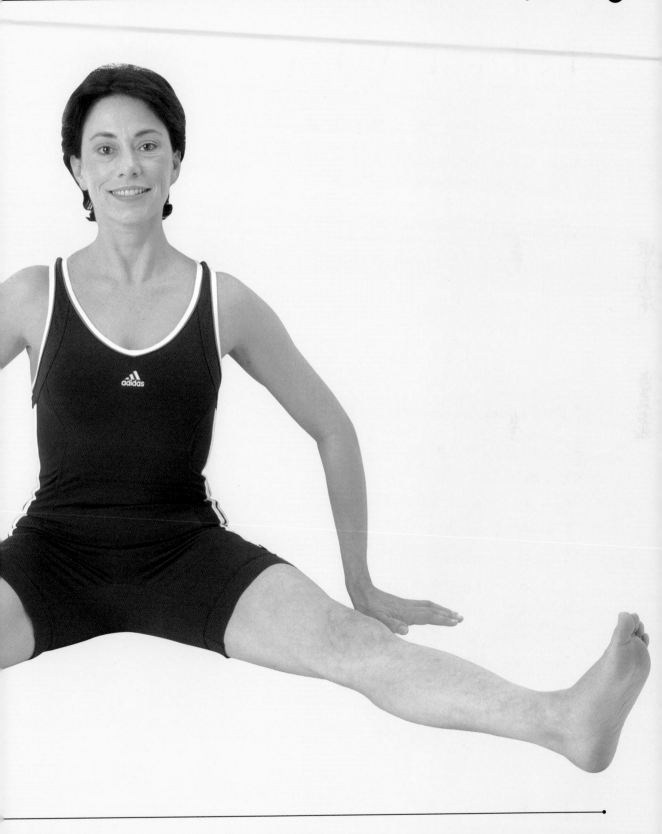

Releasing the upper body

These exercises work on the posture. The upper body is one of the three fundamental areas to be strengthened in Pilates technique (the others are the abdominals and the buttocks) and it centres on the lats and trapezius – the muscles of the back. These should also be the source of all your arm movements, rather than the shoulders themselves. As the lats and trapezius become strengthened, posture naturally improves, with the shoulders dropping down and becoming more relaxed; the chest and the ribcage opening; and the neck and head held properly and without tension.

OPENINGS – BEGINNERS

Keep your upper arms to your sides in this exercise for a wonderful feeling of opening and relaxation in your upper body.

☉ Position one

Sit on a chair or support at the right height for your knees to bend at a 90° angle. Your feet should be flat on the floor, hips-width apart, with your toes pointing straight ahead. There should be no tension in your neck or shoulders. Hold your upper arms against your sides, bending them at the elbows so they are at a 90° angle, with the palms uppermost.

☉ Position two

Breathe in and, keeping the upper arms by your sides, take your palms out to the sides so they make a semicircle around the body.

As you breathe out, return to the starting position, with your fingers pointing forwards. Repeat 10 times.

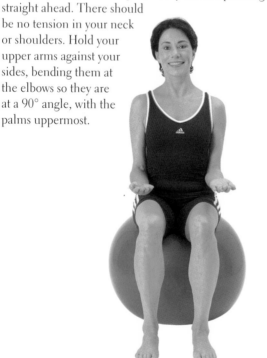

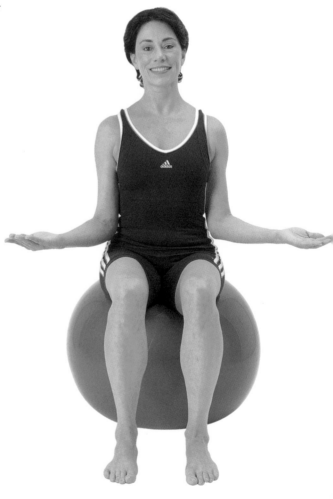

OPENINGS – ELEMENTARY

Let your arms feel as if they are carrying your breath around your body in this exercise.

➲ Position one

Sit in the same position as for the previous exercise, this time with your palms facing down.

➲ Position two

Breathe in and move your arms out to the sides, rotating them as before.

This time, when they have rotated as far as they will go, release them from your body so that your hands reach slightly outwards – only a very small gap should open up.

Breathe out to return to the starting position. Repeat 10 times.

Strengthening the back

In the studio, a series of exercises is performed using the resistance of springs to help isolate the muscles around the shoulders and so use them more effectively. You can do the same exercises at home, though, without equipment. Just make sure you feel the movement in the back first – draw the muscles down before you begin to move your arm.

UPPER BACK RELEASE – BEGINNERS

This is a small movement. Do it slowly and precisely for maximum effect.

⮌ Position one

Sit on a chair or stool close to the wall, with your feet firmly on the floor and your knees forming a right angle. Bend your arm at the elbow to make a right angle and place the back of your hand and your lower arm flat against the wall.

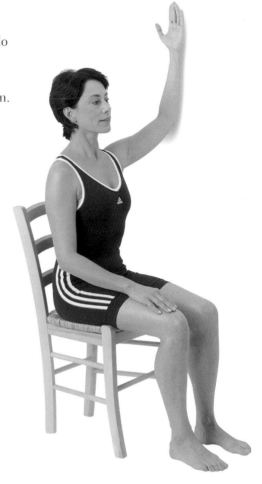

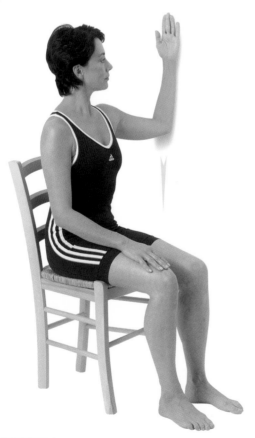

⮎ Position two

Breathe in and, as you breathe out, draw the navel towards the spine and draw your shoulder blades downwards. Let this movement in the shoulder blades draw your arm downwards, still against the wall. The movement is only one of a few centimetres but you should feel the muscles working deep inside your back. Breathe in to return to the starting position and repeat 10 times on each side.

THE COSSACK

This exercise was given as an aid to self-assessment on p. 26. Now you do it sitting down. In all these exercises, your navel is held gently against the spine, with the back straight but relaxed, and the shoulders and neck relaxed. The movement begins by drawing down the lats, the muscles below the shoulder blades, so you should feel the shoulders themselves drop as you move.

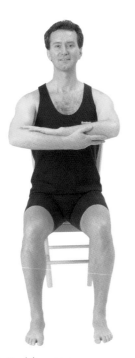

CHECKLIST

- *Check your shoulders are down and level each time you return to centre.*
- *Keep your feet firmly on the floor.*
- *Make sure your hands stay loose throughout.*
- *Don't let your hips turn to the sides as you move.*
- *Make sure there is no tension in your neck.*

↻ Position two

Breathe in deeply and, as you breathe out, begin to turn from the waist, keeping your hips facing squarely to the front. Take the turn into your upper back and let your head follow last.

Breathe in and come back to the starting position. As you breathe out, turn to the other side, then repeat 10 turns on each side in a smooth, continuous movement.

↻ Position one

Sit on a stool with your feet flat on the floor and toes pointing forwards. Fold your arms loosely, parallel with your sternum (chest). Don't grip on or hold any tension in them. Your hips should face forwards and stay in this position throughout the exercise. Draw the navel to the spine and hold it firmly throughout the exercise. Draw down the lats towards the base of your spine.

Isolating the abdominals

This first exercise is the same as the one shown earlier in the book to help you assess your posture. Here it is used as an exercise in its own right and as an introduction to a series of exercises in which you work on the movement that initiates all the pelvic tilts.

PELVIC TILTS – BEGINNERS ENGAGING

You can use this exercise to help you isolate the abdominal muscles.

⊃ Position one

Lie on your back with your feet raised on a box or a chair seat so that your knees form a right angle. Put a rolled-up towel or cushion between your thighs – this is not to squeeze, but to keep the pelvis centred through the exercise.

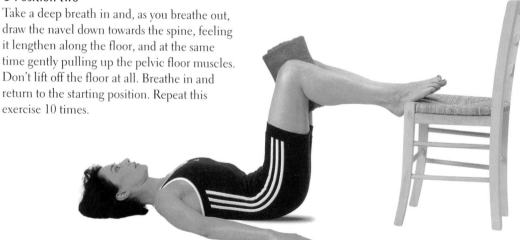

↻ Position two

Take a deep breath in and, as you breathe out, draw the navel down towards the spine, feeling it lengthen along the floor, and at the same time gently pulling up the pelvic floor muscles. Don't lift off the floor at all. Breathe in and return to the starting position. Repeat this exercise 10 times.

PELVIC TILTS ELEMENTARY – CURLING UP

Go on to this exercise only when you have located exactly which muscles you should be using, and always starting with stage one as a reminder. Don't try to curl up too high at this stage – staying in control is more important than height.

➲ Position one

Lie in exactly the same position as for the previous exercise. Breathe in deeply and, as you breathe out, draw the navel to the spine and pull up the pelvic floor.

↻ Position two

Continue to pull up the pelvic floor and draw down the abdominals so that it raises the body, vertebra by vertebra, in an arc from the floor. At the top, breathe in and curl down slowly on the out breathe. Repeat 10 times.

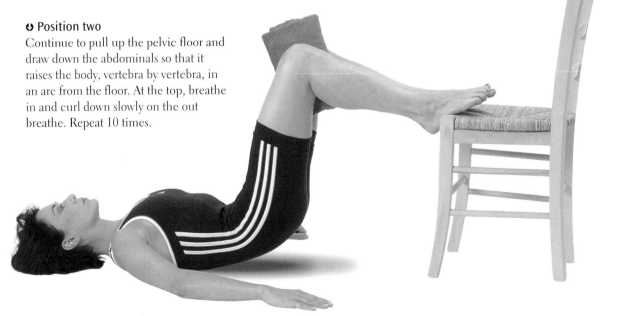

Strengthening the abdominals

Sit-ups demand a great deal of strength in the abdominal muscles if they are not to put a strain on the back. Unfortunately, many gyms and classes use sit-ups, often with a lot of repetitions, as a basic exercise without giving proper instruction on how to do them without injury to the back, and with the emphasis on how far you get up off the floor. In fact, in a good sit-up with strongly held abdominals, you come off the floor only a little way, but your abdominals curve in rather than pop out.

CHECKLIST

- *Don't expect to get your shoulders off the floor at first. In time, you will be able to get your lats off the floor but the most important factor here is that you work only the abdominals and don't let the back take any strain at all.*
- *If you feel any strain in the back, stop immediately.*
- *Don't drop the chin onto the chest. Your body should come up in a curved unit.*

SIT-UPS – BEGINNERS

➲ Position one
Lie on your back with your knees raised and a pad or book to support your head and neck. Place a rolled-up towel or cushion between your knees – this is to help activate the inner thighs, stabilise the pelvis and keep the hips square during the exercise. Your upper body should be open and relaxed – check for any tension before you begin. Place your hands on the top of your thighs.

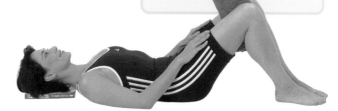

↻ Position two
Breathe in and, as you breathe out, draw the navel to the spine and activate the lower abdominal muscles. Now slowly walk your fingers up your thighs towards your knees, letting your head and shoulders curl up off the floor as they get higher. Keep the abdominals as flat as possible. If they start to pop out, you have come up too far.

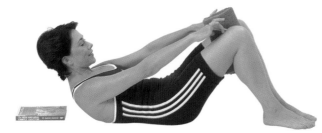

➲ Position three
At the top, breathe in and, as you breathe out, draw in your stomach muscles and roll slowly back down to the floor, sliding your fingers back down the legs.

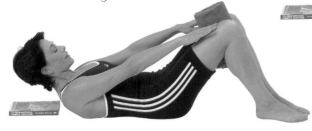

↻ Position four
When you are back in the starting position, take a deep breath and rest. Work up to 10 repeats.

OBLIQUE SIT-UPS – BEGINNERS

Oblique sit-ups work the abdominal muscles at the sides, which are just as important as those at the front. In this first exercise, don't expect to come a long way off the floor. Concentrate on becoming aware of where your oblique abdominals are.

➲ Position one

Lie on your back with your knees raised. Put a rolled-up towel or cushion between them, as in the previous exercise. Put your feet flat on the floor and your left hand behind your head. Your right arm stays flat on the floor at your side, with the palm facing downwards.

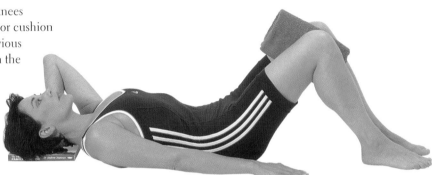

➲ Position two

Breathe in and, as you breathe out, draw the navel to the spine and activate the lower abdominal muscles. Now, using your left hand to support your head, curve diagonally, aiming your left elbow and shoulder towards your right knee. At the same time, stretch your right hand down in the direction of your feet.

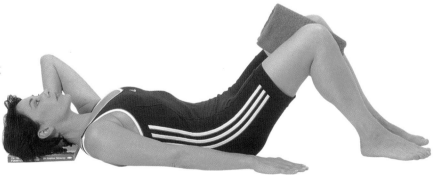

➲ Position three

Breathe in and, breathing out, draw back to the starting position. Work up to 10 sit-ups on each side.

Strengthening the central girdle

This is the first of a series of exercises that work on strengthening the abdominal muscles and correcting the alignment of the pelvis and spine. The strength of this central girdle of the body is essential to good posture and the strength of the body as a whole. It is also a vital protection for the back. Weak abdominal muscles and poor alignment will inevitably put a strain on the back and leave it open to injury.

Correct breathing helps to strengthen and protect the muscles of the back. Although your natural inclination may be to pull the stomach in as you breathe in – many people have this tendency when they try to 'stand up straight' – you should be doing the opposite. So, as you are breathing out, draw the abdominal muscles to the spine.

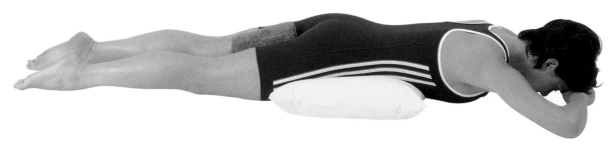

BUTTOCK SQUEEZE
This exercise is very good for locating and beginning to use the lower part of the Pilates 'girdle of strength'. You quite literally begin to get a grip on the abdominals and the muscles at the base of the buttocks.

CHECKLIST

■ *Don't let the small of the back curve in as you squeeze the rolled-up towel or cushion – keep your navel drawn towards the spine.*

■ *The upper body should be free – don't let your neck or shoulders tense up with effort.*

■ *The lower legs and feet should be relaxed – the muscles in the lowest part of the buttocks are doing the work.*

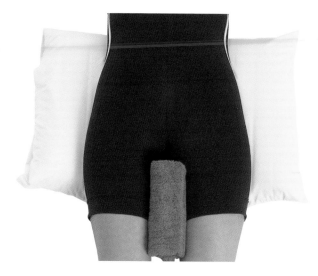

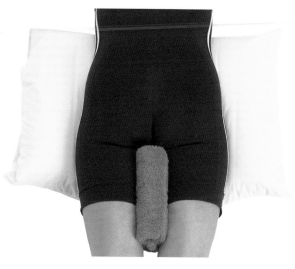

↻ Position one

Lie face down with a pillow to support your abdomen and a small cushion or rolled-up towel between your thighs. You can lie on the floor or, ideally, a hard bed so that your feet hang just over the edge. Place your head on your hands, turning it to one side if you prefer. Breathe in.

↻ Position two

As you breathe out, squeeze the towel between your thighs using the muscles at the very base of the pelvis. Try not to engage the hamstrings or the rest of the legs. Hold for approximately 5 seconds. You should feel the abdominals engage and the lower back lengthen. Release and repeat 10 times.

↻ Rest position

After you have finished the buttock squeeze, the rest position below is very good for getting rid of any strain you might feel.

From the position of the previous exercise, draw your body back so your bottom is sitting on or towards your heels. At first it is unlikely that you'll reach your heels, but just get as close as you can, taking care not to put too much pressure on your knees. Leave your arms outstretched and feel a long stretch all the way through your back. Hold this position for around 2 minutes.

> ### A BIGGER STRETCH
>
> *As you become looser you will find that you can manage to sit on your heels. To help you stretch, ask a friend to put one hand at the top of your back and the other in the small of your back, and push their hands apart gently. This extends the stretch and feels wonderful!*

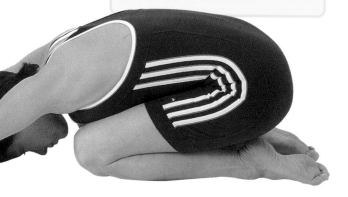

Toning the legs

These exercises are the first in a series that stretch and strengthen the leg muscles from the buttocks right down to the feet. The alignment of the body is very important if you want the legs to work properly, so many of these exercises are performed with your back against a wall – ensuring that shoulders and hips stay square. It is also vital that your leg is in the correct position before you begin any of the exercises – if you can, it's a good idea to set up a mirror to check your positioning and to ensure you're parallel.

A FLAT BACK

In this exercise, it is very important to keep your back supported against the wall with your hips facing directly forwards. This will keep your legs parallel.

OUTER THIGHS – BEGINNERS
This exercise creates a very pleasing hollow in the outer thigh rather than that all-too-common bulge.

➲ Position one
Lie on your side with your back supported against a wall. Let your lower arm stretch out, and place a pillow or a folded towel, between this arm and your head. It is also a good idea to place a small cushion or folded towel beneath your waist, as this gives support and reminds you not to let your waist fall in. Bend your lower leg and place your straight upper leg on a large, firm cushion or two. Flex the foot of your upper leg and place your left hand on your hip to stabilise the pelvis.

☽ Position two
Take a deep breath in and, as you breathe out, draw the navel to the spine and the lats down into your lower back. Your waist lengthens, creating a long, low lift in the upper leg with the hip, knee and flexed foot facing forwards.
This is first and foremost a stretch – but the stretch is so strong that it turns into a leg lift. Lower and repeat 10 times on each leg.

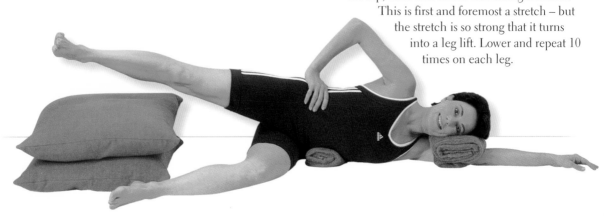

INNER THIGHS – BEGINNERS

The muscles of the inner thighs are often completely forgotten. This exercise will help you to locate and strengthen them.

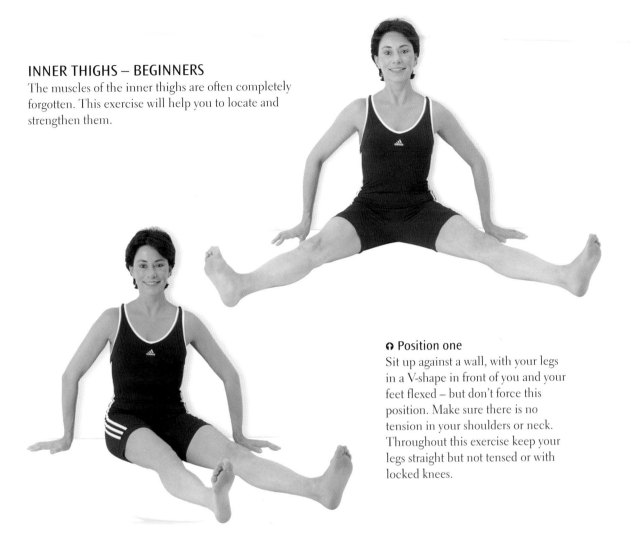

⌒ Position one

Sit up against a wall, with your legs in a V-shape in front of you and your feet flexed – but don't force this position. Make sure there is no tension in your shoulders or neck. Throughout this exercise keep your legs straight but not tensed or with locked knees.

⌒ Position two

Breathe in and, as you breathe out, move your right leg slowly towards the left, keeping the foot flexed and without letting your pelvis move away from the wall. You should feel the muscle of your right inner thigh working. Move your right leg back to its starting position and then move your left leg towards the right in the same way. Alternate, 10 times on each leg.

ADDING A WEIGHT

If you have difficulty feeling this movement in your upper thigh, place your hand on the inside of your leg and exert a slight pressure so that you have to work a little harder.

As you get stronger, you can use a weight to increase the effort. Put an ankle weight on the floor just to the side of your leg, so that the leg has to push it across the floor – this is actually more effective than strapping the weight to the leg.

REMEDIAL LEGS

These exercises were originally developed for specific hip and knee joint problems or injuries in the legs, hence the name. However, they work just as well as ultra-safe strengtheners for the leg muscles.

BEGINNERS

For the best results, do this exercise as slowly and mindfully as possible. When your leg is fully extended but still supported, you should feel muscles engaging immediately above your knee.

↻ Position one

Lie back on the floor with your head and shoulders leaning against a firm cushion and most of your spine on the floor. Bend your right leg over a large folded cushion, keeping your left leg bent.

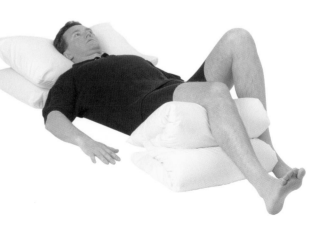

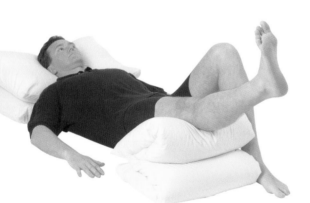

↺ Position two

Breathe in and, as you breathe out, draw in the abdominals, flex your right foot and raise it so that the leg extends out from the knee. Feel as if a piece of string is attached to your big toe and is pulling you up. Don't lift the leg off the cushion but feel it extend fully.

↪ Position three

Return to the starting position and repeat with 10 slow lifts on each leg.

REMEDIAL LEGS – ELEMENTARY

Again, do this exercise slowly, putting as much movement in the foot as you can.

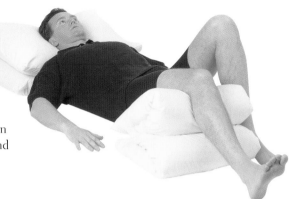

➲ Position one

Lying in exactly the same position as for the previous exercise, extend your right leg as before, with the foot gently flexed.

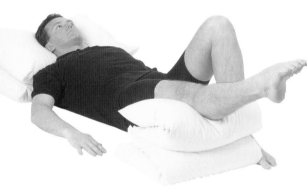

↺ Position two

When your leg is fully extended, point the toe slowly and firmly. Don't let your knee or ankle bend. Your foot should be in one long straight line from your leg. Hold this position for a few seconds.

➲ Position three

Now flex your foot back, feeling the stretch through the back of the knee. Lower your foot to the floor and repeat the sequence 10 times for each leg.

Toning the arms

All of these exercises will strengthen and tone the arm muscles. Later, as the arms become stronger, you can add weights but for now concentrate on becoming aware of the muscle groups that you are using.

ARMS – BEGINNERS
➲ Position one
Lie on your back with your knees lifted, and your feet flat on the floor a hip-width apart. Check that your spine is not hollowed out or pressed into the floor, and that your neck and shoulders are relaxed. Place your arms in a rounded shape in front of you, with your hands level with your sternum (chest).

CHECKLIST

■ *Imagine you are holding a beach ball in front of you so that your arms retain a wide curve throughout the exercise.*

■ *The movement begins with the hands level with the sternum (chest). Do not allow them to move up to shoulder or chin level, as this can cause tension.*

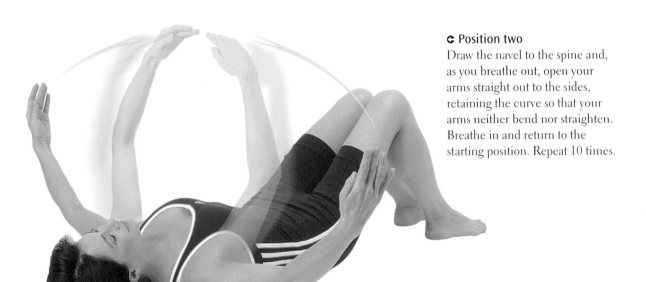

↻ Position two
Draw the navel to the spine and, as you breathe out, open your arms straight out to the sides, retaining the curve so that your arms neither bend nor straighten. Breathe in and return to the starting position. Repeat 10 times.

ARMS – ELEMENTARY

This exercise works the triceps, the muscles at the back of the upper arms. The breathing pattern is not as important in these two arm exercises – just make sure you don't forget to breathe.

↻ Position one

Lie on your back with your knees raised, your feet on the floor and your arms stretched straight up towards the ceiling. Now place your left hand behind your right elbow as a support.

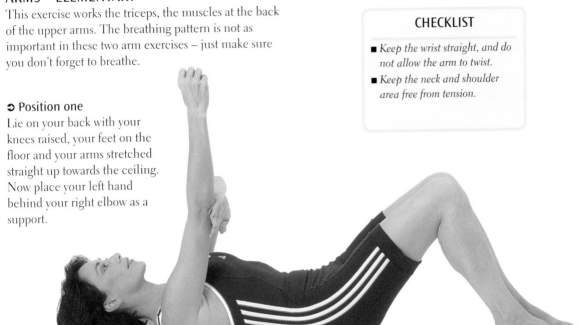

↻ Position two

Lower your right hand slowly towards your right shoulder, then make a fist and bring it back up in one slow movement. Repeat 10 times and then change arms.

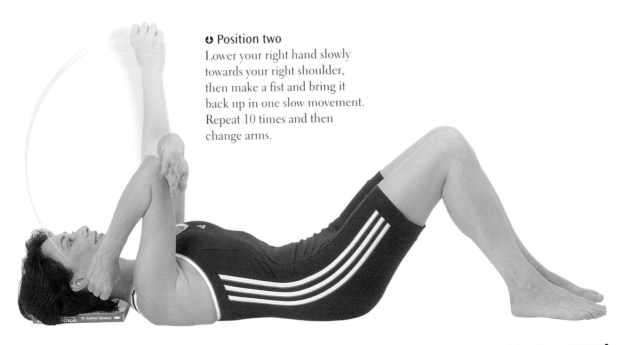

Inner thigh squeeze

Pilates technique uses a series of cushion squeezes. You will
need a cushion that is quite hard so that you need to exert
considerable pressure to squeeze.

CUSHION SQUEEZE – BEGINNERS
↻ **Position one**
Lie on your back with your knees bent
and your feet flat on the floor. Your arms
should be down by your sides, relaxed.
Check that there is no tension in your
shoulders or neck, and that your back is
in a relaxed, neutral position. Place a
cushion between your thighs.

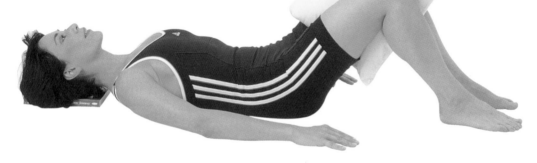

↻ **Position two**
Breathe in and, as you breathe out,
draw the navel to the spine and squeeze
the cushion in a long, slow movement
to the count of ten. Make sure your
pelvis does not lift off the floor. Release
and repeat up to 10 times.

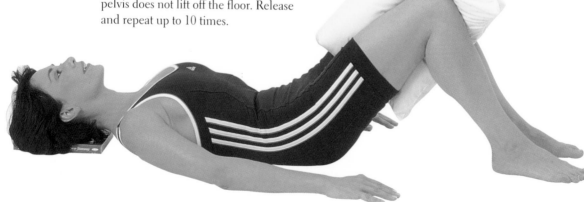

THE CAT

This is a wonderfully sinuous exercise where the aim is to get the movements to flow seamlessly into each other. If you have any back problems only do positions one and two.

⊃ Position one

Position yourself on your hands and knees – if you can, do this sideways on to a mirror so that you can check that your back has a natural curve. Your knees should be a hip-width apart so that your shoulders, hips and knees are aligned.

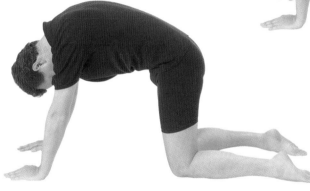

↻ Position two

Breathe in and, as you breathe out, draw your navel to your spine. Dropping your head down, arch all the way through your back. Breathe in to return to the starting position, with a flat back.

⊃ Position three

This time, as you breathe out, reverse the movement so that your head and your bottom are the highest points, with your back scooped down in a bowl shape. Breathe in and return again to the starting position. Repeat up to 10 times.

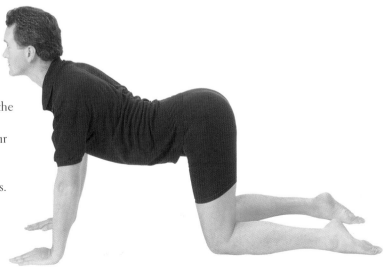

The Pilates Workout: level two

Words of Wisdom

'Limber and stretch muscles and ligaments ... your body will be as supple as that of a cat, not muscular like that of a brewery-truck horse.'
JOSEPH PILATES

When you feel confident that you can perform all of the exercises in level one correctly and comfortably, without any straining, you are ready to move on to level two.

At this point, the exercises become more complex. You are working several parts of the body simultaneously and so you need to concentrate on using all of the muscle groups properly, as you learnt at the first level. The key to this is to perform the exercises slowly.

You will also start to use weights. There are two sorts of weights needed – ankle weights and hand weights (dumb-bells). The ankle weights are widely available from sports stores and you simply wrap them around your ankle, where indicated in the exercises. If you have dumb-bells or you intend to buy them, they should weigh 1kg. However, you can just as easily use ordinary food cans – hold one in each hand, unless instructed otherwise.

What you have achieved so far

■ *You have started to work at the slow, rhythmic Pilates pace and developed deep, even breathing.*

■ *You have isolated the muscles to be used during your programme and learnt to use them with precision and control.*

■ *Your posture will be improving and you should be losing stored tension.*

Your goals for level two

■ *Build on the exercises of level one to tone your muscles further.*

■ *Work on strengthening key areas, including with the use of weights.*

■ *Improve all joint mobility and, in particular, increase suppleness in the back.*

Again, it is important to give
yourself plenty of time on this level
before going on to the final, advanced
programme. Do all of the exercises
slowly and thoroughly, feeling each
group of muscles working at the
deepest level.

Some of the exercises from level
one are repeated in the programme for
level two. Begin with the warm-ups (see
pp. 46–57), and then go on to work on
the upper body.

Releasing the upper body

In all of these exercises, the navel is held gently against the spine. Your back should be straight and your neck and shoulders relaxed. Always begin the movement by drawing down the lats.

SHOULDER SHRUGS WITH WEIGHTS

This exercise is the same as the one in the warm-up (see p. 54) but now it is done with weights to help you really stretch out the arms and work the lats. Here, you can drop the shoulder shrugs from your warm-up.

(see p. 54)

CHECKLIST

- *Keep your shoulders and neck relaxed as you press back.*
- *If your neck and shoulders tense up, try the movement without weights.*
- *Make sure you are breathing deeply and rhythmically, to prevent tension.*
- *Your arms should be straight but not tense throughout the exercise.*

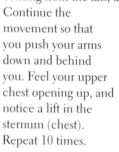

⟳ Position three

Relax your shoulders as you breathe out and pull them right down, with the movement coming from the lats, deep into the back. Continue the movement so that you push your arms down and behind you. Feel your upper chest opening up, and notice a lift in the sternum (chest). Repeat 10 times.

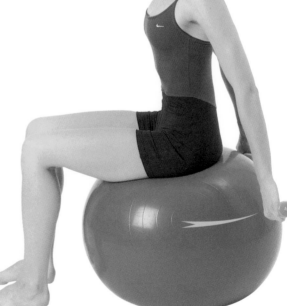

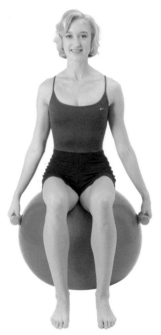
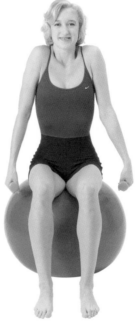

↻ Position one

Sit on a chair or support, preferably facing a mirror, with your feet flat on the floor and facing forwards. Let your arms hang down, relaxed at your sides, holding a 1kg weight or can in each hand.

↻ Position two

Now, breathe in and lift up your shoulders towards your ears. Keep your arms long – don't bend them at the elbow.

CLOCK FACE

This is an exercise for the lumbar region of the back – rather like a lumbar and sacral massage. The 'clock face' does not refer to the circle that the knees are making but to the circle of the lumbar region.

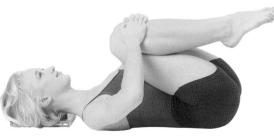

↶ Position one

Lie on your back, with the whole spine gently stretched out along the floor, your knees drawn up to your chest and your feet relaxed. Place your hands just below your knees.

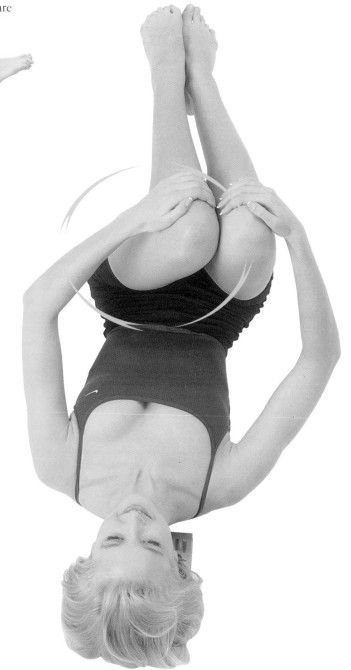

↷ Position two

Breathe in and, as you breathe out, draw in the abdominals and keep them drawn in throughout the exercise. Now, with the hands guiding your knees, describe a very small circle with your knees, but concentrate on the larger circle that your back is making on the floor. Don't let your hips tip, and keep the movement deliberately slow and small. Trace 10 circles clockwise, then 10 anti-clockwise.

Releasing the upper spine

This is the first of two exercises that are very good for people who tend to store tension in the shoulders, back or neck. It opens up and loosens this whole area which, in turn, helps to improve the breathing.

USING THE TOWEL

This exercise uses a rolled-up towel. Take an ordinary hand towel and roll it up tightly, then secure both ends with elastic bands. However, if the towel feels too uncomfortable, try the exercise without it.

UPPER BACK RELEASE – BEGINNERS
↻ **Position one**
Lie on your back, with your knees raised and the feet flat on the floor. Place a rolled-up towel beneath the middle of your shoulder blades and stretch your arms straight up in the air, fingertips pointing at the ceiling and palms facing forwards, but without tension.

↻ **Position two**
Breathe in and, as you breathe out, draw the navel to the spine and take one arm straight back so that the upper arm is next to your ear. At the same time, take the other arm forwards so that it lies against your side, with the fingers pointing down towards the toes. Breathe in again, and, as you breathe out, reverse the position of the arms. Alternate arm movements, breathing deeply, 10 times.

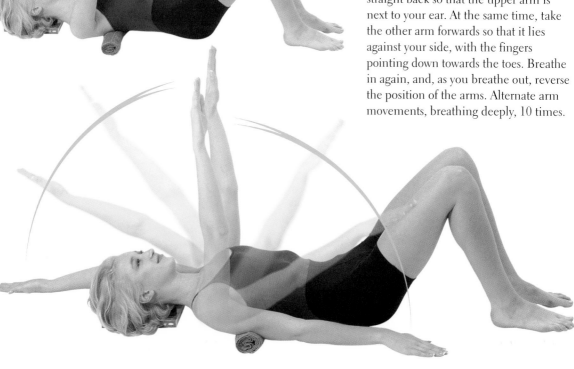

HIP ROLLS – ELEMENTARY

This is a more advanced version of the hip rolls in the warm-up. Here, however, the feet are apart. This gives you a much greater stretch, which you should feel all the way across your body.

⊃ Position one
Lie on your back with your feet and knees in line with your shoulders and your neck and spine long and relaxed. Bend your arms and place both hands beneath your head.

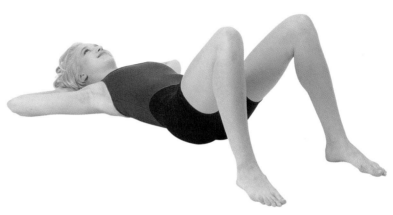

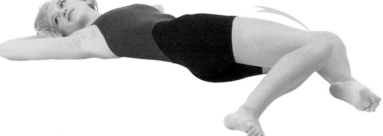

↺ Position two
Breathe in and, as you breathe out, roll your knees towards the floor. If your lower knee can reach the floor easily, try to get the other knee down too. As you stretch, let your head roll in the opposite direction to your knees so that the oblique stretch goes right through the body.

⊃ Position three
Breathe in to return to the starting position, then, breathing out, stretch in the opposite direction. Alternate smoothly from side to side, 10 times on each side.

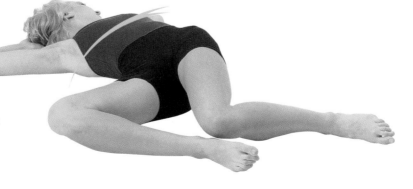

Mobilising the lower back

Incorrect use of muscles can lead to lower back pain and stiffness. These exercises help release any accumulated tension in this all-important area.

PELVIC TILTS – INTERMEDIATE

This is the third stage of the pelvic tilt, and now arm movements are added to the exercise. However, before you do this, repeat the first two stages (pp. 64–65) as a preparation.

⮌ Position one
Breathe out, drawing the navel to the spine, and pull up the pelvic floor.

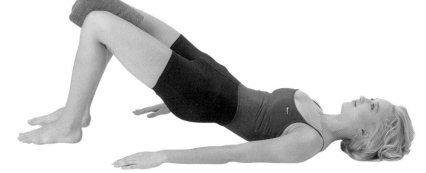

⮌ Position two
Start to curl your hips slowly off the floor, keeping the navel drawn towards the spine.

⮌ Position three
When your body has curled up as far as it can comfortably go with the abdominals still held in, breathe in and start to raise your arms.

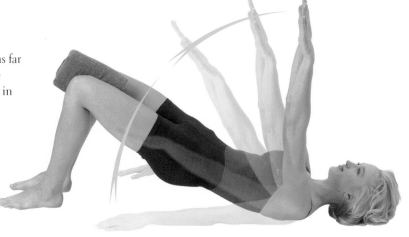

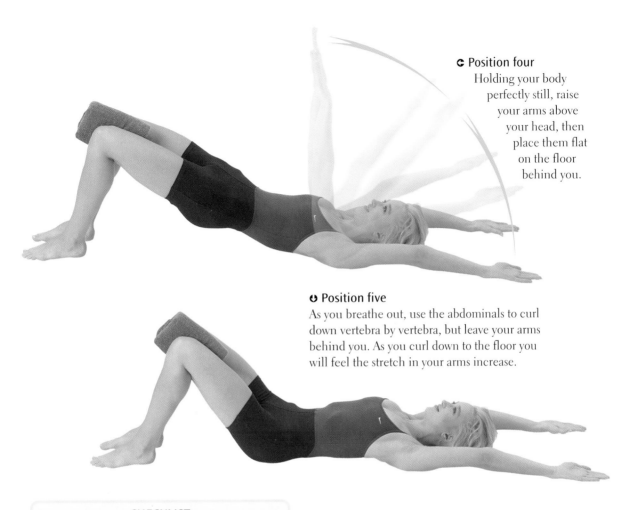

↻ Position four
Holding your body perfectly still, raise your arms above your head, then place them flat on the floor behind you.

↺ Position five
As you breathe out, use the abdominals to curl down vertebra by vertebra, but leave your arms behind you. As you curl down to the floor you will feel the stretch in your arms increase.

CHECKLIST

■ *Make sure you breathe correctly – breathing is a vital part of this exercise.*

■ *Try to isolate the vertebrae more each time you repeat the exercise. Ideally, your back should become as sinuous as a snake.*

■ *Don't let any tension get into your shoulders, chest or neck. If they do start to tense, you are coming too far off the floor.*

■ *Always begin by drawing the navel towards the spine and engaging the pelvic floor muscles for a moment before you start to move off the floor.*

■ *The more slowly you do these pelvic tilts, the more effective they are.*

↺ Position six
Breathe in again and lower your arms to your sides. Repeat 10 times, the slower the better.

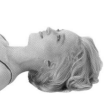

Strengthening the central girdle

The following exercises are the next steps in the series that began with the buttock squeeze (see p. 68), which you should repeat 10 times before going on to these exercises.

HEEL LIFTS

After you have completed the buttock squeeze, remove the cushion from between your thighs for this exercise.

↻ Position one

Lie in the same position as for the buttock squeeze, checking that your abdominal muscles are engaged and that your neck and shoulders are relaxed. Hold this position throughout the exercise.

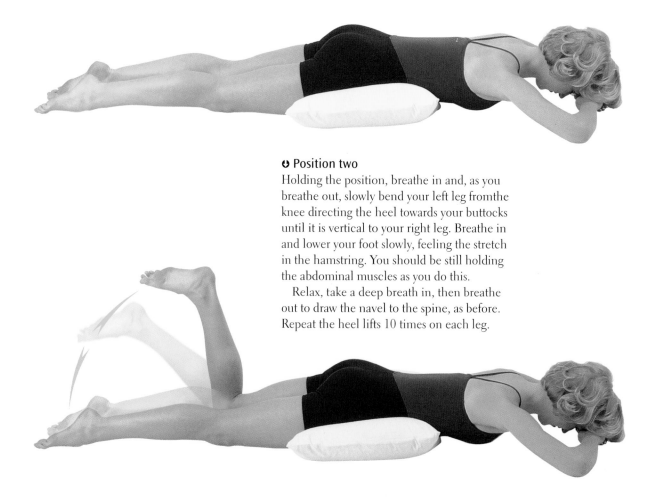

↻ Position two

Holding the position, breathe in and, as you breathe out, slowly bend your left leg from the knee directing the heel towards your buttocks until it is vertical to your right leg. Breathe in and lower your foot slowly, feeling the stretch in the hamstring. You should be still holding the abdominal muscles as you do this.

Relax, take a deep breath in, then breathe out to draw the navel to the spine, as before. Repeat the heel lifts 10 times on each leg.

PREPARATION FOR THE ARROW

The arrow is one of the most in-depth exercises for the whole central girdle, and is presented in full on p. 110 in level three. This introductory exercise strengthens the muscles that will be used.

↻ Position one

Lie in the same position as for the previous exercise, but this time with your arms stretched out above your head.

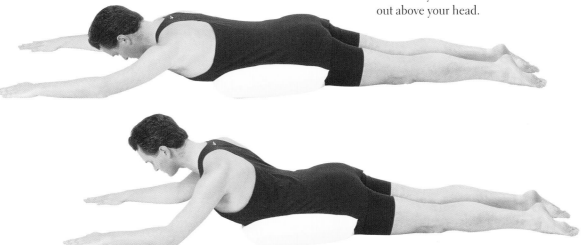

↻ Position two

Breathe in, then breathe out as you draw down the lats and trapezius muscles so that the arms are also drawn down and your head and chest lifts up slightly, in line with the spine. Lower and repeat, working up to 10 repetitions.

↻ Position three

Spend a few moments in the rest position (see p. 69).

CHECKLIST

- *Don't try to lift your upper body far from the floor – this is essentially a long, low stretch.*
- *Make sure your abdominal and buttock muscles are engaged throughout. Rest if you feel tired.*

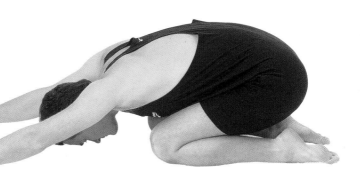

Toning the legs

Your legs should now be feeling stronger and you should be much more aware of their various muscles groups. The exercises on the next four pages work on strengthening, toning and stretching the legs further.

SIDE LIFTS

In this exercise, the leg lifts further than in the exercise on p. 70. Keep checking that your knees, feet and hips are all parallel and facing forwards.

↻ **Position one**
Lie on your side, with your back supported against a wall, your hips parallel and facing forwards, and with a small rolled-up towel supporting your waist. Place a folded towel or cushion between your head and your lower arm. Place your other hand on the floor in front of you for support.

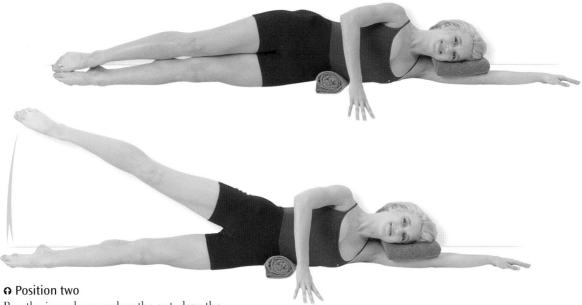

↻ **Position two**
Breathe in and, as you breathe out, draw the navel to the spine and raise the top leg with the knee facing forwards. You should be able to feel the muscle working all the way up the thigh. Lower and repeat 10 times on each leg.

↻ **Position three**
When you can raise one leg with ease, you can do a double leg lift. Keep the lift low (it is a much harder exercise to do) and stop if you feel a strain. Work slowly up to 10 repetitions.

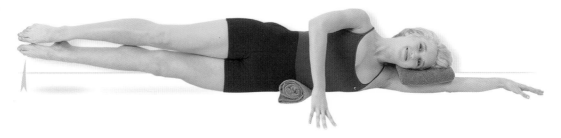

INNER THIGHS – ELEMENTARY

The next two exercises strengthen the muscles of the inner thigh, which are often forgotten. You are using the same muscles as in the exercise on p. 71. If you have difficulty isolating the correct muscles, repeat the earlier exercise.

↻ Position one

Lie on your side with your back supported against a wall. Make sure your hips and shoulders are in line – keep them next to the wall throughout the exercise, even when your legs are moving. Put a rolled-up towel or big cushion in front of you and rest your top knee on it. Rest your head on your lower arm and stretch the straight lower leg away from you.

↻ Position two

Breathe in and, as you breathe out, extend your lower leg with your foot gently pointed. Keeping the knee facing squarely forwards, lift your heel slowly and as high as possible. Breathe in as you lower it. Try to make the whole movement smooth. Repeat for 10 lifts each side.

FEELING STRONGER?

This exercise repeats the movements of the previous one but this time with the addition of ankle weights. Don't go on to this until you can do the exercise effortlessly, without using weights.

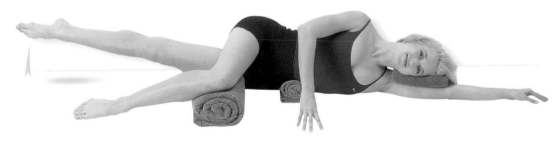

OUTER THIGHS – ELEMENTARY

This exercise repeats the one in level one (see p. 70) but now you use an ankle weight.

↻ Position one

Strap on ankle weights and lie on your side with your back supported against a wall. Let your lower arm stretch out and place a folded towel, or pillow folded double, between this arm and your head with another smaller towel to support your waist. Bend your lower leg and place your upper leg on a large, firm cushion. Flex the foot of your upper leg and place your upper arm on your hip.

(see p. 70)

CHECKLIST

- *Keep your back supported against the wall with the hips facing directly forwards.*
- *Keep your legs parallel.*
- *The slower the movement and more stretched out the leg, the better it is.*

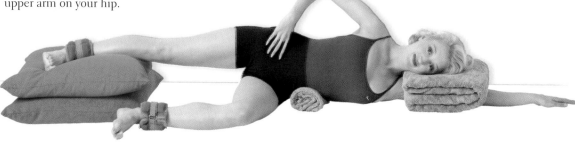

↻ Position two

Breath in and, as you breathe out, lengthen your top leg away from your pelvis, and lift it as high as possible while maintaining a parallel position – press your hip down with your right hand to stabilise the pelvis during this exercise. Breathe in to lower your leg. Repeat 10 times on each side.

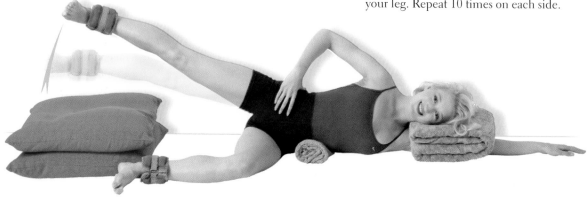

GLUTEAL STRETCHES

There are two stages of this stretch for the gluteal muscles of the buttocks, the first one being easier. It is also a diagonal stretch for the back.

BE GENTLE

- *Don't force the turn. If you feel any strain in the back, stop immediately.*
- *Make sure that the hand on your right leg is on the thigh, not the knee.*

STAGE ONE
↻ Position one

Sit on the floor with your legs straight and your right hand supporting you. Cross your right leg over your left with the knee raised, and the right foot behind your left knee.

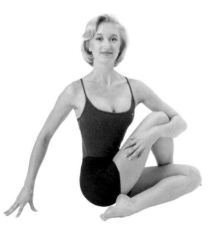

↺ Position two

Turn smoothly to the right. Feel the stretch starting in the buttocks and going through the upper body until your head turns. Hold the stretch then return to the starting position. Repeat 4 times on each side.

STAGE TWO
↻ Position one

For the next stage, sit up and bend the left leg, bringing the foot towards the buttock. Cross your right leg over your left, placing your left hand on the raised thigh.

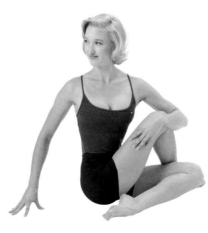

↻ Position two

As before, turn towards the supporting hand in a slow, smooth, controlled movement, feeling the stretch move gradually through your body. Keep your back upright.

Strengthening the abdominals

The abdominal muscles are central to balance, strength and posture – but that strength can take some time to acquire. Take these exercises very gently and stop if you see the abdominals start to bulge out. This means you are putting too much strain both on the abdominal muscles and those in the back, and you are probably trying to take the movement further than is safe just yet. The oblique abdominals are the muscles you feel when you twist or bend.

SIT-UPS

Only go onto these sit-ups when you can do those in level one with ease (see p. 66–67). Nothing is accomplished by straining to come up a long way – it just makes your abdominal muscles bulge out and puts a strain on your back. It's better to keep the movement smaller and more controlled.

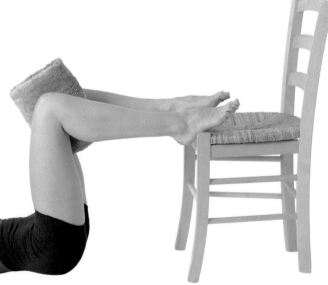

♁ Position one

Lie on your back with your feet on a chair so that your knees form a right angle. Place a rolled-up towel or cushion between your knees. Place your hands behind your head. Check that your shoulders and neck are relaxed.

♃ Position two

Breathe in and, as you breathe out, draw the navel to the spine and curl your head and shoulders off the floor, keeping the chin dropped and the shoulders and neck relaxed. Don't struggle to sit all the way up. It's much more important that the abdominals are still in a scooped-in shape; if they start to bulge out or quiver you have come up too far. Return slowly, rolling down to the starting position. Repeat the exercise 10 times.

OBLIQUE SIT-UPS

The oblique abdominals are likely to be under-developed compared to the central ones, so don't attempt to come off the floor too far at first.

↻ **Position one**
Lie on your back with your knees raised. Place your left hand behind your head and your right on top of the abdomen, so you can feel whether the abdominal muscles are working properly.

↻ **Position two**
Breathe in and, as you breathe out, draw the navel to the spine and the lats down your back. Now curl over towards your right as if you were getting out of bed. Think of your left elbow aiming towards your right hip. When the oblique abdominal muscles are really strong, the aim is to get the whole of the lats off the floor – but very few people manage this. Come up only as far as the abdominal muscles can hold without bulging or quivering. Lower and change sides, working up to 10 repeats on each side.

SINGLE LEG STRETCHES

This (and the double leg stretch, see p. 120) are two of the best-known original Pilates exercises. The names are somewhat misleading as they both entail a great deal more work than a simple stretch of the leg.

(see p. 120)

CHECKLIST

- *Hold your basic position – navel to spine, and head and shoulders curled up – throughout the exercise. Don't lie down fully until you have finished.*
- *Start with the extended leg higher off the floor. As you become stronger you can lower it towards the floor.*

⟳ Position one

Lie on your back and draw your knees to your chest. Keep your knees shoulders-width apart, with the feet touching. Draw the navel to the spine and curve the upper torso forwards as you slide your hands down to your ankles.

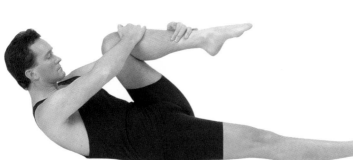

⟲ Position two

Breathe in and, as you breathe out, stretch out your right leg and draw your left knee to your chest, keeping your left hand on the left ankle. This helps to keep your ankle in line with your knee.

⟳ Position three

Breathe in, then breathe out as you stretch. Change legs so that this time the left leg is stretched away from you. Alternating, repeat 10 times on each leg.

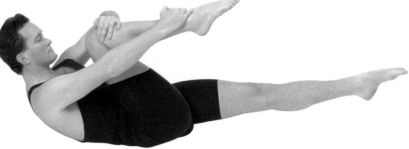

Strengthening the arms

These exercises will strengthen and tone the arm muscles. Practise first without weights, then as your arms become stronger, you can add the weights. You can use dumb-bells (up to 1kg) or simply use food cans held in the hands.

CHECKLIST

- *Hold your arms in a wide curve throughout.*
- *Always start with your hands level with the sternum; avoid the tendency to hold them much higher up towards shoulder level.*

ARM WEIGHTS – BEGINNERS

This exercise was done in level one without weights – if your arms still find this a strain, continue as before.

↻ Position one

Lie on your back with your knees lifted, feet flat on the floor hips-width apart. Check that your back is supported against the floor, and your neck and shoulders are relaxed. Let your arms form a rounded shape with the hands level with the sternum (chest). If you are using weights, hold one in each hand.

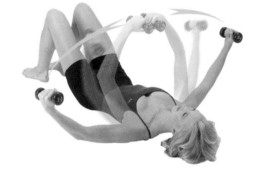

↻ Position two

Breathe out, draw the navel to the spine and open your arms out to the sides, retaining their curved shape. Breathe in and return to the starting position. Repeat 10 times.

ARM WEIGHTS – ELEMENTARY

This is a new exercise, so try it without weights to start with, and ensure that you keep the arms curved throughout.

↻ Position one

Lie on your back, as in the previous exercise, with your arms in an oval shape in the air. If you are not using a weight, clasp your fingers loosely together. If you are, hold just one weight in both hands.

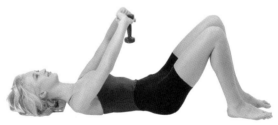

↺ Position two

Breathe out to draw the navel to the spine and take your hands back behind your head, keeping your arms in an oval. Don't go too far or the abdominals will bulge out. Breathe out to return to the starting position, and repeat 10 times.

Strengthening the back

This exercise is for the muscles of the back, which are often neglected or completely forgotten. You need to do this exercise very slowly, focusing all of your attention on your back so that you become fully aware of these muscles.

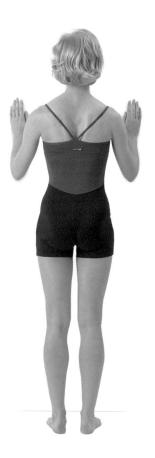

↻ Position one
Face a wall with your toes almost touching it. Your feet should be hips-width apart. Ensure your back is straight and there is no tension in your neck and shoulders. Place your palms flat on the wall at shoulder height.

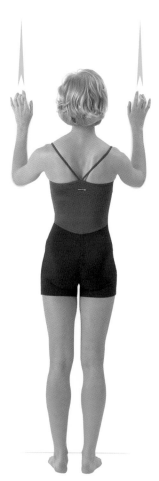

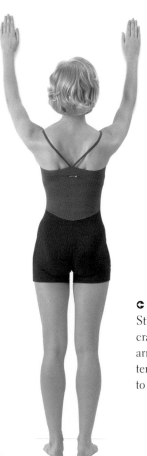

↷ Position two
Breathe in and crawl your fingers very slowly up the wall. As your hands move gradually upwards, feel the separate muscles that are being used within your back.

↻ Position three
Still breathing in, continue the crawling movement until your arms are outstretched but without tension. Do not lift your shoulders to get higher.

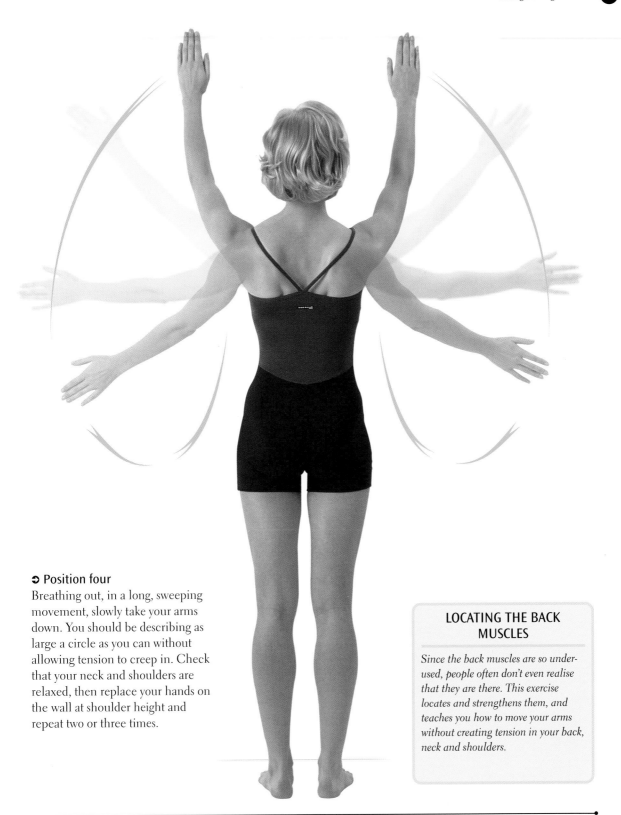

↪ Position four

Breathing out, in a long, sweeping movement, slowly take your arms down. You should be describing as large a circle as you can without allowing tension to creep in. Check that your neck and shoulders are relaxed, then replace your hands on the wall at shoulder height and repeat two or three times.

LOCATING THE BACK MUSCLES

Since the back muscles are so under-used, people often don't even realise that they are there. This exercise locates and strengthens them, and teaches you how to move your arms without creating tension in your back, neck and shoulders.

Working the legs

REMEDIAL LEGS – INTERMEDIATE

This is the third stage of the remedial leg exercises and now includes a turn-out. Remember, turn-out always originates in the hip socket, not the leg or foot. Before you do this exercise, repeat the first two in the series (pp. 72–73). Do no worry if your breathing pattern does not match the movements just as long as you do not hold your breath in.

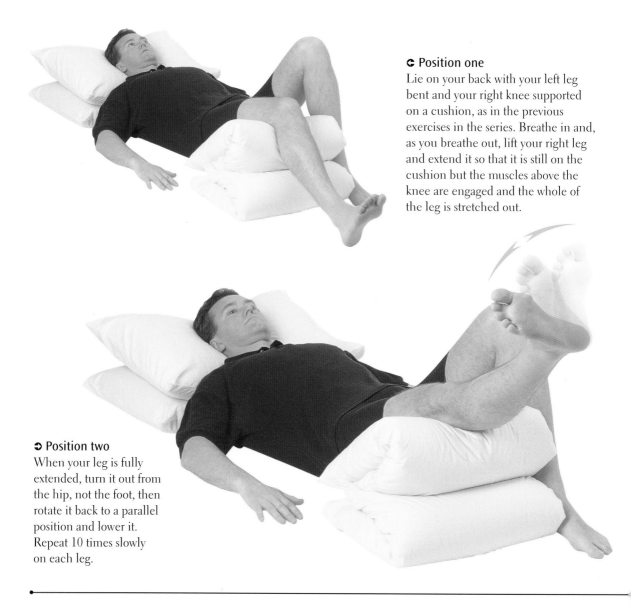

↻ Position one
Lie on your back with your left leg bent and your right knee supported on a cushion, as in the previous exercises in the series. Breathe in and, as you breathe out, lift your right leg and extend it so that it is still on the cushion but the muscles above the knee are engaged and the whole of the leg is stretched out.

↪ Position two
When your leg is fully extended, turn it out from the hip, not the foot, then rotate it back to a parallel position and lower it. Repeat 10 times slowly on each leg.

QUAD STRETCH

You will feel this exercise as a strong stretch all the way up the front of the thigh. You need to find a strong, stable surface such as a table or a kitchen counter to take your weight.

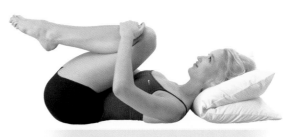

⮰ Position one

Sit on the very edge of the table, then lie down with a cushion to support your head and neck, and your knees drawn gently up to your chest.

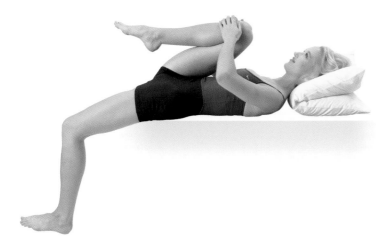

⮲ Position two

Draw the navel to the spine and make sure the whole of your back is in contact with the table. Let your left leg hang down over the edge of the table, while you hold the right leg gently to the chest, keeping the abdominals engaged and your entire back on the table. Hold the position for at least 3 minutes. The weight of the overhanging leg will stretch out your thigh muscles and the front of your hip.

⮰ Position three

Keeping the abdominal muscles firmly engaged and your back in contact with the table, change legs. Repeat 4 times with alternate legs keeping a natural breathing pattern throughout the exercise.

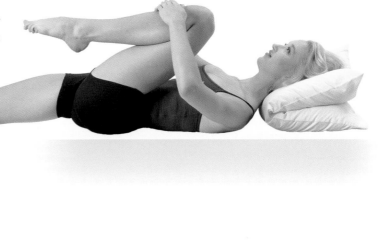

HAMSTRING STRETCH

The hamstring muscles are often very tight, particularly in women who wear high-heeled shoes. Do not force the stretch – just take it as far as you need to in order to feel a stretch, but not a strain.

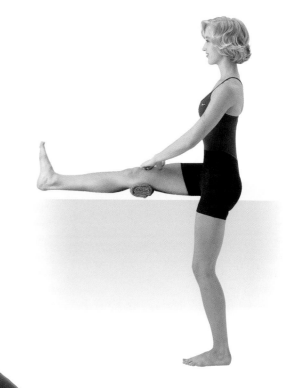

↪ Position one

Sit on the edge of a bed or table, with one leg straight out in front of you resting on the surface and the other foot on the floor – make sure your hips are square. Place a rolled-up towel or small cushion under-neath the knee of the stretched leg and flex your foot. Make sure your back is straight and you pull the navel back towards the spine.

↩ Position two

Breathe in and, as you breathe out, lean your upper body forwards smoothly, keeping your foot flexed. You will feel the stretch in the back of the leg, in the hamstring. When you reach the limit of your stretch, hold it for a few seconds. This is a slow, gentle stretch, so do not reach forwards too far. Breathe in and return to the starting position. Repeat 10 times on each side.

CHECKLIST

■ *Don't try to bounce this stretch to increase it – it is a single, slow movement.*

■ *If you feel any strain in your back, stop immediately.*

CUSHION SQUEEZE – ELEMENTARY

This cushion squeeze is much harder than the one in level one, and you will feel it very strongly in the inner thigh muscles. Do the cushion squeeze on p. 76 as a warm-up for this one.

RELAX

Since this exercise requires a lot of effort, it is very easy for tension to creep in. Between each squeeze, check your neck, arms, back, shoulders and even your face. Relax and repeat.

↻ Position one

Lie with your back completely flat on the floor and your legs straight and stretched out in front of you. Place a firm cushion between your feet, which should be gently flexed.

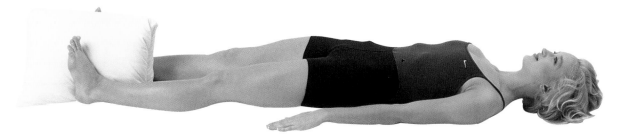

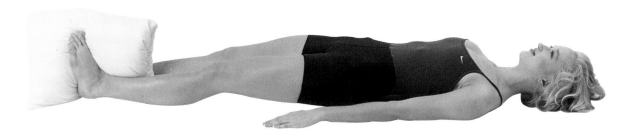

↻ Position two

Breathe in and, as you breathe out, draw the navel to the spine and engage the pelvic floor muscles. Now squeeze the cushion between your feet. You should feel the whole length of the inner thigh muscles working. Release, and repeat 10 times.

The Pilates Workout: level three

When you can perform all of the exercises of levels one and two with ease, you are ready to go on to the final stage of Pilates exercises in level three.

Don't feel you have to rush into doing this. It is much better to spend more time strengthening the muscles than to attempt to do exercises that your body isn't quite ready for, and so won't be able to do correctly. The whole of the central girdle – lats, abdominals, buttocks – need to be very strong for some of these exercises, especially those like the advanced sit-ups, the arrow, the dog or the double leg stretches.

It is still very important to prepare the body before such exercises, so always do the warm-up first and spend time on these deceptively simple exercises; they are the foundation for all of the more difficult ones.

What you have achieved

■ *You will by now have seen a very noticeable improvement in your muscle tone and strength.*

■ *Your posture will be more centred and graceful, and your limbs will be moving with less effort and more precision.*

■ *You will have increased mobility and suppleness.*

Your goals for level three and beyond

■ *Further muscular strengthening and toning, particularly of the central girdle.*

■ *Improved coordination within more complex exercises.*

■ *A sense of posture and placement that becomes natural poise in all daily movements.*

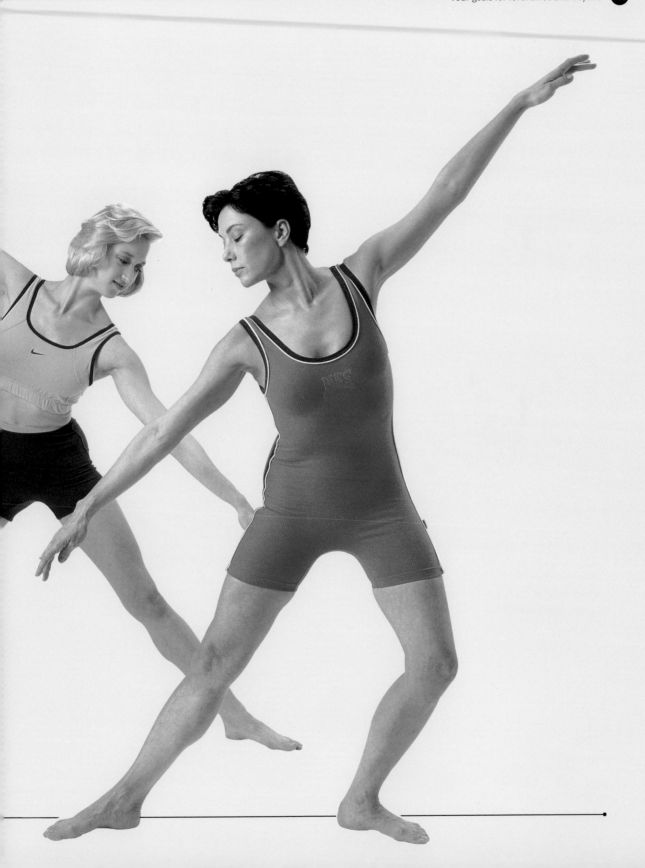

Releasing the spine

This exercise will be a good release for you if you have a tendency to store tension in the shoulders, back or neck. It follows on from the first upper back release (p. 62), opens up that whole area and improves the breathing.

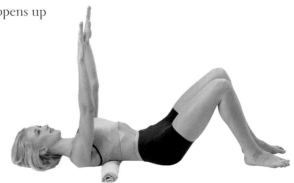

UPPER BACK RELEASE – ELEMENTARY
⮎ Position one
Lie on your back with your knees raised and a rolled-up towel supporting your upper back. In this exercise, the arms describe an entire circle. Begin with the arms raised and your fingers pointing up to the ceiling.

⮎ Position two
Breathe in and, as you breathe out, draw the navel to the spine and take one arm back behind your head and one forwards on the floor, with your fingers pointing to your toes.

⮎ Position three
Breathing in, rotate your arms out to the sides, simultaneously, until they are both at 90° to the body.
  Now turn the palms over and breathe out to continue the circle until your arms have changed positions.

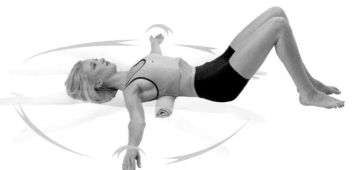

⮎ Position four
Breathing in, bring both arms back to the starting position, then begin again with the other arm going back first. Alternate for 10 repetitions.

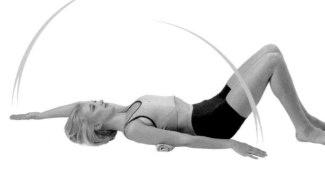

UPPER BACK RELEASE – INTERMEDIATE

This exercise extends the arm and back movements used in the earlier versions on pp. 60–61. As before, make sure you are using your back muscles rather than your shoulders.

➲ Position two
With your upper arms against your sides, begin to open the chest by moving your hands and lower arms slowly outwards.

↻ Position one
Sit on a chair, with your knees bent at right angles, and your shoulders even and relaxed. Bend your arms at the elbows, keeping the upper arms to your sides and the palms facing downwards. In this exercise the movement is more important than your breathing – breathe naturally.

➲ Position three
Now lift your upper arms away from your sides and gently pull your elbows behind your torso. Don't lift your shoulders.

↻ Position five
To release the back, wrap your arms around your chest, drop your head, and draw the navel to the spine as you breathe out. Repeat 10 times.

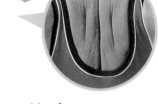

↻ Position four
Extend your arms behind you as far as they will go without distorting or lifting the shoulders. Feel the squeeze in your back as the shoulder blades push together.

Mobilising the spine

This is the final stage of the pelvic tilts and, as its name implies, the most advanced. It is a difficult movement and not one that should be tried until the abdominals are strong. As with the previous exercises, begin with a deep breath and, as you breathe out, draw the navel to the spine, draw up the pelvic floor and curl the spine off the floor in a smooth curve. Begin with some of the more basic pelvic tilts (see pp. 64–65, 84–85) as a warm-up.

> ### IMPORTANT
>
> *This strenuous exercise is particularly tough on the abdominal muscles. Do each position properly rather than going through the sequence 10 times immediately. If you get any pain in your back, or if your stomach starts to bulge out or quiver, stop at once. In this exercise, work to coordinate you breathe with the movement.*

PELVIC TILTS – ADVANCED
Ɔ Position one
Lie on your back with your knees raised, your feet flat on the floor and your arms, neck and back relaxed. Put a rolled-up towel or cushion between your thighs.

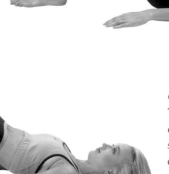

Ɔ Position two
Take a deep breath in and, as you breathe out, draw the navel down towards the spine, draw up the pelvic floor and slowly curl your back away from the floor.

Ɔ Position three
When your body has curled up as far as it can comfortably go with the abdominals still held in, breathe in and lift your arms up above your head and place them flat on the floor behind you.

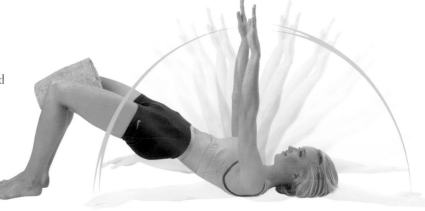

↻ Position four

As you breathe out, curl down vertebra by vertebra, not forgetting to use your abdominal muscles and leaving your arms behind you. As your spine curls down to the floor, you will feel the stretch in your arms increase.

➲ Position five

Breathe in, place your hands very gently beneath your head and, as you breathe out, raise your upper body very slightly off the floor, with your nose pointing straight up to the ceiling.

➲ Position six

Now, continue to breathe out and curl forwards so your head faces forwards and you feel the curve reach the middle of your ribs.

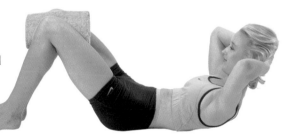

↺ Position seven

Finally, still breathing out, release your hands from behind your head and stretch them towards your knees, so that the movement is felt in the lower abdominal muscles. Breathe in as your return to position one. Build up to 10 repetitions, resting when necessary.

The girdle of strength

The following exercises extend the work of the heel lifts in level two (see p. 80), making the lifts harder each time. However, only add weights or the rolled-up towel when you are completely comfortable with the basic exercise. If you feel you are taking the strain in the back, remove the weights at once.

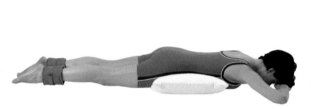

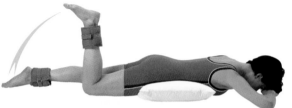

HEEL LIFTS – ADVANCED
ↄ Position one

Strap on ankle weights and lie on your front with a pillow beneath the abdomen and your face resting on your hands. Check that your abdominal and pelvic floor muscles are engaged and that your neck and shoulders are relaxed. Remember to hold this position throughout the exercise.

ↄ Position two

Holding the position, breathe in and, as you breathe out, slowly bend your lower leg from the knee as far as it will go in the direction of the buttocks, or until it is vertical with the floor. Make sure your heel does not move from the centre line. Breathe in and lower your foot, still holding the position. Repeat 10 times for each leg.

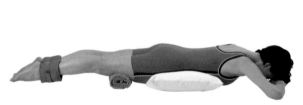

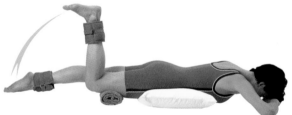

HEEL LIFTS WITH TOWEL
ↄ Position one

Do this exercise first without weights but avoid it altogether if you have a knee injury or feel any strain. Lie face down with a pillow under the abdomen. Place a rolled-up towel under your legs, just above your knee. Rest your face on your hands and keep the upper body as relaxed as possible.

ↄ Position two

Breathe in and, as you breathe out, draw the navel to the spine, engage the lower buttock muscles and hold this position throughout the exercise. Slowly bend your lower leg from the knee following the instructions from the previous exercise. Lower and repeat 10 times, then repeat 10 times on the other leg.

STOMACH STRETCHES

For this exercise to work properly, you need to keep the stomach and pelvic floor muscles engaged throughout. Start with just one or two repetitions, building up to five as you feel stronger.

↻ Position one
Lie face down, with your arms and legs stretched out, hands and feet hip-width apart, palms down and legs turned out with the feet pointed. Use a pillow under the stomach and hips to support your lower back.

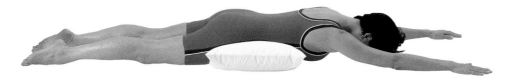

➲ Position two
Breathe in and, as you breathe out, keeping stretch in your arms and legs, lift your left arm and your right leg approximately 5cm (2in) off the floor.

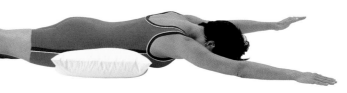

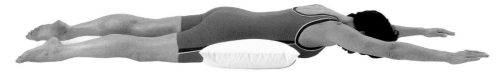

↻ Position three
Breathe in to lower. Breathe out and repeat with the right arm and the left leg.

➲ Position four
Breathe in and, breathing out, lift both arms and legs 5cm (2in) off the floor. Repeat the whole sequence 5 times.

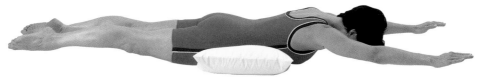

THE ARROW

The Arrow uses every area of the central girdle – the lats, the abdominal muscles and the buttocks all work in unison. Always start with the buttock squeezes and the heel lifts (pp. 68–69 and 86–87) before you practise The Arrow, so you can check that all your muscles are working to their maximum before you start.

↻ Position one

Lie face down on a hard bed or on the floor with a cushion beneath your abdomen. Place a pillow beneath your forehead so that you can look down comfortably. Put your arms by your sides, with your fingers pointing to your feet.

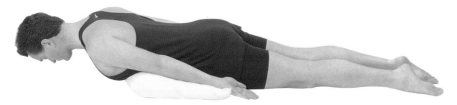

⟳ Position two

Breathe in and, as you breathe out, engage the abdominal, pelvic floor and buttock muscles. Lift your arms towards the ceiling, pull the shoulder blades down towards the pelvis, and lift your sternum (chest) and head away from the floor. Keep your head facing the floor.

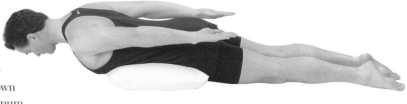

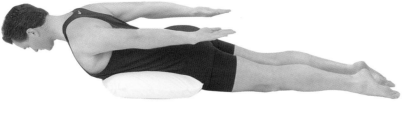

↻↺ Position three

Neither your arms nor your upper body should come high off the floor; this is a long stretch rather than a lift. Hold the lift for approximately 4 seconds. Breathe in to come down, and repeat 10 times.

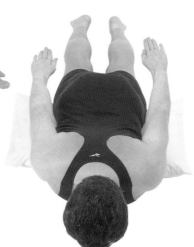

REST POSITION WITH HELP

After The Arrow, take a short rest. This rest position
is an extension of the one in level one. If you are
working with a partner, you could ask for help with this
stretch. Ask your partner to place one hand at each end
of the spine and pull the hands gently further apart.

CHECKLIST FOR THE ARROW

- *Don't try to come up too far from the floor.
  This is really a long two-way stretch.*
- *Keep your palms facing the ceiling.*
- *Don't let your neck or shoulders tense.*
- *Keep your arms straight but not stiff.*
- *Breathe very slowly and deeply.*

⮌ Position one

From the Arrow position, draw your
body back so that you are sitting on
your heels with your arms stretched
out in front of you.

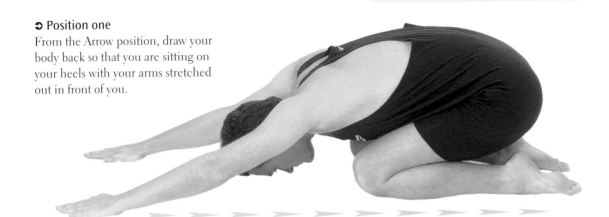

⮌ Position two

Bring one arm down and place it
next to your side with your fingers
pointing to the toes. Then bring the
second arm down to your side – you
may find it more comfortable to let
your head roll to one side. Stay like
this for a few moments and relax,
breathing deeply.

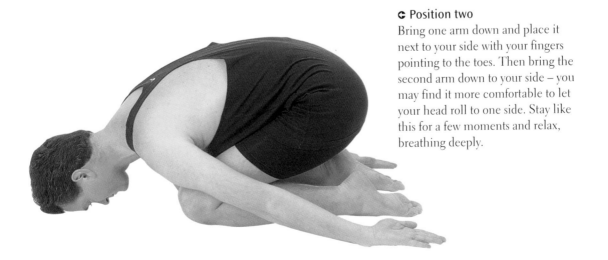

Releasing the back

In this third stage of the hip rolls, we show the exercise with arms outstretched. However, you may find it helpful at first to hold on to a heavy piece of furniture. Position it behind you so you can hold on with your arms behind your head. The legs of a heavy chair or table, about 60–90cm (2–3ft) apart, would be ideal.

HIP ROLLS – INTERMEDIATE
⊃ Position one
Lie on your back with your arms extended out to the sides or holding onto a piece of furniture to steady yourself. Make a right angle with your knees so that your thighs are vertical and your calves are parallel to the floor.

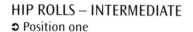

⊂ Position two
Breathe in and, as you breathe out, keeping your knees together, stretch them slowly to one side, feeling an oblique stretch across the body. The movement should start in the top buttock for maximum stretch.

⊃ Position three
You will have to let your hips come off the floor but your shoulders should stay down. Your head should turn in the opposite direction from your legs each time. Alternate for 10 slow rolls each side.

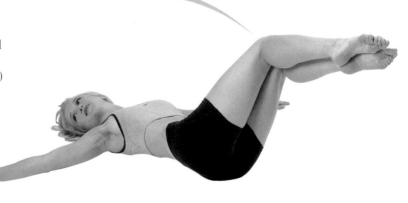

HIP ROLLS – ADVANCED

When you can do the previous exercise comfortably, try this exercise. It requires even more strength in the abdominals as they have to sustain the weight of the whole leg.

↻ Position one
Lie on your back as in the previous exercise, using a piece of furniture to anchor you if you wish, or with your arms stretched out to the sides. Your legs should be stretched out on the floor.

⊃ Position two
As you breathe in, bend your left knee slowly and draw it up towards your chest, keeping your foot pointed. Keep your right leg stretched out on the floor.

↻ Position three
Roll your left leg, still bent, across to the right. Turn your head to face the opposite direction.

⊃ Position four
Stretch the leg and let its weight drop it gently towards the floor. Leave it there for a moment, feeling the stretch. Breathe in, bend the leg, and use your stomach muscles to roll back to the centre, bringing your knee back to your chest. Breathe out and slowly straighten the leg back to the starting position. Change legs and repeat the exercise on the other side. Alternate 10 times on each side.

SIDE TWIST

This exercise combines a side stretch with a twist. It open up the sides of the body and works on the waist – but you must be careful to keep your hips completely still while you are doing it.

WATCH YOURSELF

Do this exercise in front of a mirror if you can. This will help you keep checking your posture and position. In particular, watch that your back stays straight, your shoulders stay down and your hips remain parallel all the way through.

⮌ Position one

Sit up straight, with your legs stretched out in front of you. Bend your left leg so that the foot is level with the right knee. Allow your left knee to drop towards the floor. Raise your arms above your head, fingers pointing towards the ceiling.

⮌ Position two

Stretch out your spine, keeping your neck and head in alignment. Breathe in and move your torso smoothly round to face your bent knee, keeping your hips parallel.

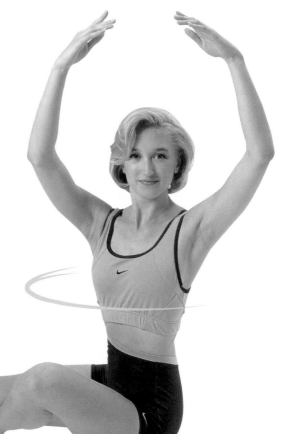

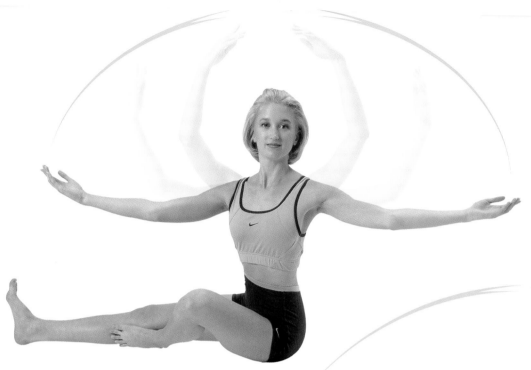

↷ Position three
Lower your arms straight out to the sides. Your palms should be facing the ceiling, and your hips should not have moved. Check that your shoulders are relaxed, and your back and chest are open.

↪ Position four
Breathe out and curve your body smoothly down towards the straight leg, bringing the upper arm in a long overhead curve, with the lower arm reaching towards the inside of the foot. Hold the stretch for a few moments, if you can.

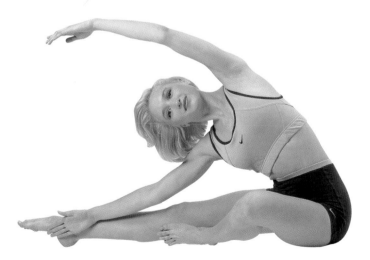

↩ Position five
Breathe in, turn parallel to face your outstretched foot and stretch out along the leg. Return to the starting position and repeat four times on each side.

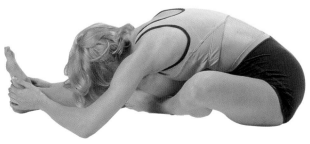

Toning the legs

The first exercise is a repeat of previous ones but is now made harder by using ankle weights. Keep checking that the knee, foot and hips are all parallel and facing forwards, for the full benefit from this exercise. The second exercise, rondes de jambes, is based on ballet *barre* work but, because you are lying down, it ensures that you stay in alignment, which can often get distorted if you are standing at the *barre*. It demands a great deal of strength in the abdominals, as well as in the legs.

OUTER THIGHS – INTERMEDIATE
↻ Position one
Strap on your ankle weights. Lie on your side, with your back supported against a wall, your hips parallel and facing forwards, and with a small rolled-up towel to support your waist. Place your hand on your hip and gently press down towards the floor. This will ensure the work is concentrated on the outer thigh.

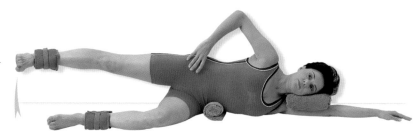

↻ Position two
Breathe in and, as you breathe out, draw the navel to the spine and raise the top leg with a gently flexed foot, and the knee facing forwards. You should be able to feel the muscle working all the way up the thigh.

↻ Position three
Raise your leg to its full extent, checking with your hand that the hip stays parallel and doesn't shift. Lower, and repeat 10 times on each leg.

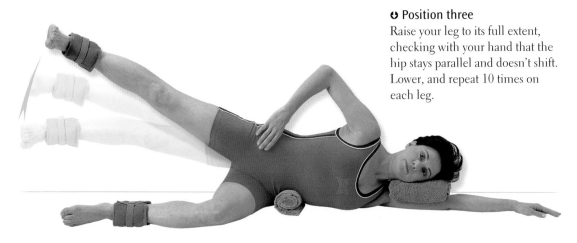

RONDES DE JAMBES

Literally, this means 'leg circles', but the circle is very small, traced with the toe.

◑ Position one

Lie on your side with your back supported against a wall, your hips parallel, a rolled-up towel under your waist and your top hand on your hip. Bend your top leg at a right angle in front of you. Stretch your lower arm out, resting your head on it.

↻ Position two

As you breathe out, raise your lower leg. It will not be able to come very far off the ground.

↻ Position three

Now, rotate from the hip so the leg is turned out and point the foot.

Describe four circles with your toe, clockwise and anti-clockwise. Repeat 10 times with each leg.

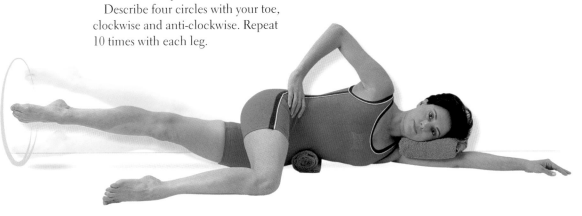

Strengthening the abdominals

When you can do the sit-ups from level two with ease (see pp. 92–94), you can make it harder by changing your position so that your feet are on the floor, with your knees raised up, instead of resting on a chair. This way, you have further to go.

SIT UP – ELEMENTARY
⤴ Position one
Lie on your back with your knees raised and your feet flat on the floor. Put your hands behind your head. Check that your shoulders and neck are relaxed.

⤸ Position two
Breathe in and, as you breathe out, draw the navel to the spine and lift your head and shoulders off the floor, keeping your chin dropped and your neck and shoulders as relaxed as possible.

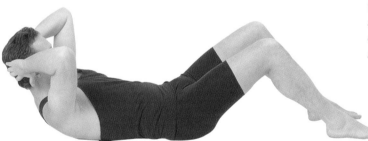

⤴ Position three
Breath in, then breath out and try to deepen the curve and raise the upper torso further forwards, stretching your arms towards your knees. Don't struggle to sit all the way up – it is more important that your abdominals remain in a scooped-in shape. If they start to bulge or quiver you have come up too far. Hold the curve, place your hands back behind your head and return slowly to the starting position, rolling down. Repeat 10 times.

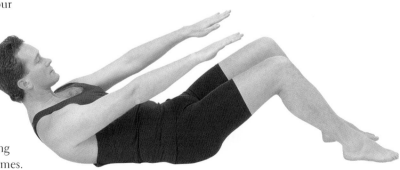

THE OBLIQUE STRENGTHENER

This exercise works the oblique abdominal muscles and trims the waist. Begin with positions one and two and go on to position three only when you can do the first part comfortably.

↻ Position one

Lie on the floor with your knees bent, your spine straight and the navel pressing lightly towards the spine. Put your right arm straight on the floor by your side and bend your left arm at the elbow, with the hand lightly holding your head.

STABILISER

To help you hold this position easily and to keep your knees in place, put a rolled-up towel or cushion between your knees as a stabiliser. You could also tuck your feet under a piece of furniture or ask a friend to hold them in place

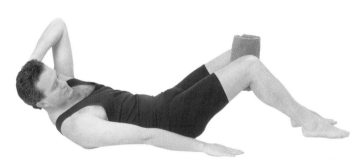

↺ Position two

Breathe in and, as you breathe out, reach your right arm towards the right thigh and curve your upper torso up from the floor, without straining or tensing the shoulders. As you come off the floor, stretch your left elbow and shoulder towards your right knee.

↻ Position three

Holding the body in place, use the abdominal muscles to raise your right arm.

↺ Position four

Breathe in and stretch your left arm across the body, placing your left palm over your right. Breathing out, stretch both arms beyond the right knee. Now place your left hand back behind your head and return to the starting position.

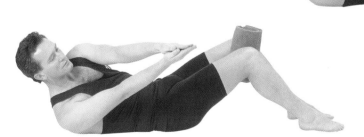

DOUBLE LEG STRETCH

Before doing the double leg stretch, it is a good idea to do 10 single leg stretches from p. 94 (5 on each leg) as a warm-up. This is a strenuous exercise, so don't expect to be able to do 10 repetitions to start with – just do 3 or 4 well, and work up gradually.

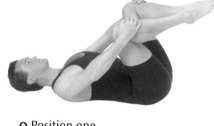

➲ Position two

Breathe in and, as you breathe out, draw the navel to the spine, keeping your tailbone on the floor. Curl your head and shoulders up off the floor, with your chin down towards, but not on, your chest.

↻ Position one

Lie on the floor with your back flat and your knees bent up towards your chest, shoulder-width apart. Place your hands just below the knees and check that your neck and shoulders are relaxed.

↻ Position three

Breathe in and stretch out your arms and legs, together, so that they are at an angle of 60° to the floor. Turn out the legs, squeezing your inner thighs together.

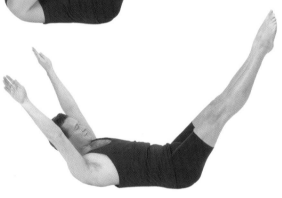

↻ Position five

As you breathe in, continue the circle of the arms out to the sides and then up towards an angle of 60° again. Point your toes.

Breathing out, slowly bend both your knees and elbows, place your hands just below the knees, and rest your head and upper back on the floor. Repeat the whole sequence up to 10 times.

↻ Position four

Keeping your legs and feet where they are, breathe out and stretch your arms up to the ceiling, then back behind your head, brushing past the ears. Turn the palms out.

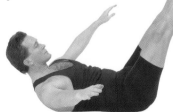

THE DOG

This exercise has some similarities to The Cat (see p. 77) – but it requires a lot more strength and a good sense of balance.

(see p. 77)

⮂ Position one

Begin in the same position as The Cat, with the weight evenly distributed between your hands and knees, your feet hips-width apart and your back in a natural positions – not too flat.

⮂ Position two

Breathe in, and gently arch your back as you curl your right elbow and left knee towards one another under the torso. You are now balancing on your left hand and right leg.

↻ Position three

Now, breathe out and extend your right arm and left leg and stretch them out fully, keeping them parallel with the floor.

Repeat the exercise at least 5 times, then change arms and legs and repeat 5 times on the other side.

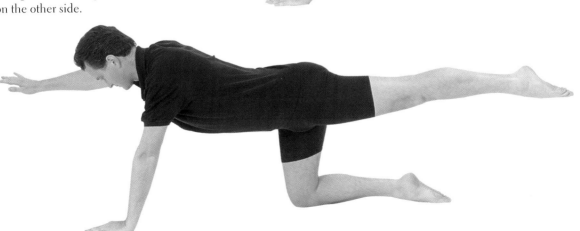

Releasing the upper body

Begin with the four upper body exercises to centre yourself
and to release tension in the neck, back or shoulders. Start
with the shoulder shrug with weights (p. 80), then the two
openings (pp. 60–61 and 105) and then The Cossack (p. 63).

ARMS AND LATS

The following exercise for the upper body builds on
the exercises already done and stretches out the lats
even more. For this exercise, you will need a short pole
(about 60–90cm, 2–3ft long) or a rolled-up towel,
secured with elastic bands.

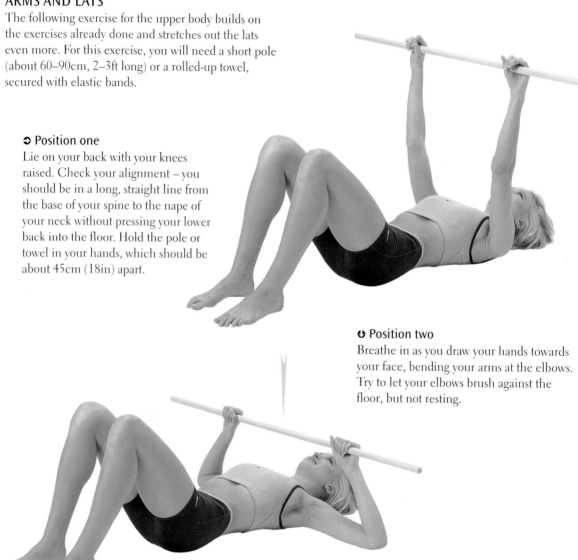

⤴ Position one

Lie on your back with your knees
raised. Check your alignment – you
should be in a long, straight line from
the base of your spine to the nape of
your neck without pressing your lower
back into the floor. Hold the pole or
towel in your hands, which should be
about 45cm (18in) apart.

↻ Position two

Breathe in as you draw your hands towards
your face, bending your arms at the elbows.
Try to let your elbows brush against the
floor, but not resting.

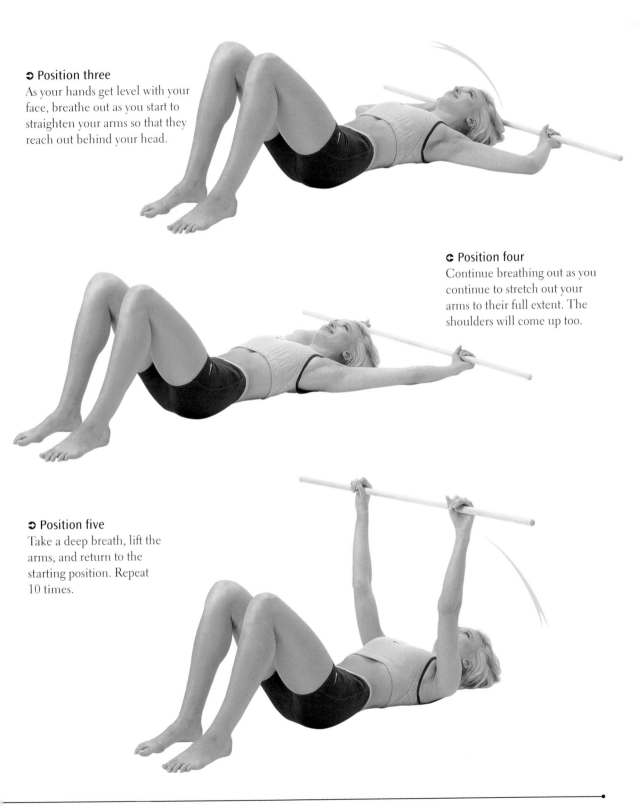

➲ Position three
As your hands get level with your face, breathe out as you start to straighten your arms so that they reach out behind your head.

↩ Position four
Continue breathing out as you continue to stretch out your arms to their full extent. The shoulders will come up too.

➲ Position five
Take a deep breath, lift the arms, and return to the starting position. Repeat 10 times.

Strengthening the arms

Continue with the arm exercises from level two using weights but now add these ones, too (see p. 95). If your arms feel the strain, begin without weights to make sure you are moving correctly, and only add the weights as you become stronger. Do not worry too much about the breathing pattern – you can change it to suit your own rhythm.

ARMS – INTERMEDIATE
↻ **Position one**
Lie on your back with your knees raised and your arms stretched straight up towards the ceiling. Hold a weight in your left hand. Now place your right hand behind your left elbow, as a support.

↺ **Position two**
Breathe in and, as you breathe out, draw the navel to the spine. Slowly lower your left hand (with the weight) towards your left shoulder.
    Then bring it back up in a slow movement into the air. Repeat 10 times, and then repeat on the other side.

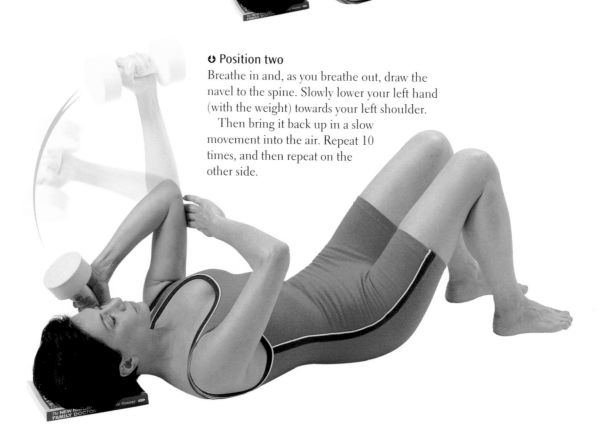

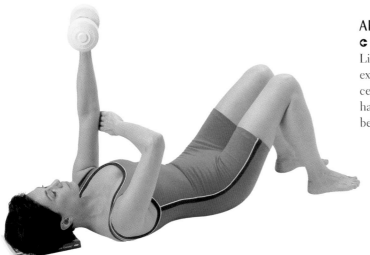

ARMS – ADVANCED
↻ Position one
Lie on your back as in the previous exercise. Stretch your arms up to the ceiling, holding a weight in your left hand only. Place your right hand behind your left elbow, as a support.

↺ Position two
Breathe in and, as you breathe out, draw the navel to the spine. Slowly lower your left hand (with the weight) – but this time, taking it across towards the right shoulder.

Bring it back up in a slow movement into the air. Repeat 10 times on each arm.

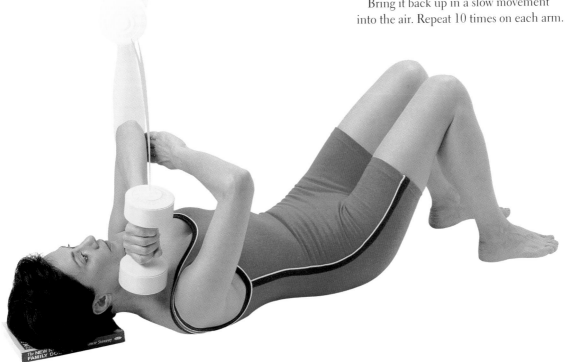

ARM EXERCISES – STANDING

Here are some more arm exercises, this time in a standing position. It is very important that you start from a secure stance so that you can concentrate on what your arms are doing and not put any strain on your back.

DELTOIDS

The deltoids are the muscles on top of the upper arms. To work these muscles completely, repeat Position one with your arms in front of the hips and Position two with your arms behind the hips – about 10cm (4in) in each direction. Strengthening the deltoids will help to improve posture, particularly rounded or hunched shoulders, as well as making your joints more mobile.

↻ Position one

Stand about 30cm (1ft) away from a wall, with your back to it. Place your feet hip-width apart so that your shoulders, hips and knees are all in line. Bend your knees slightly and let your entire back lean against the wall.

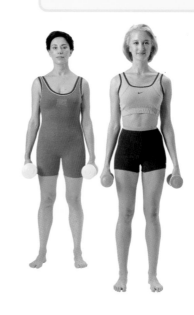

↺ Position two

Breathe in and, as you breathe out, press down the lats and begin to raise your arms.

Lift both arms straight up to the side, until they are at right angles to the body. Take care not to lift your shoulders. Lower and repeat 10 times.

TRICEPS AND BICEPS

The triceps and biceps are both muscles used in your everyday arm movements. The biceps are at the front and the triceps at the back of the upper arm. This next exercise tones and firms this whole area.

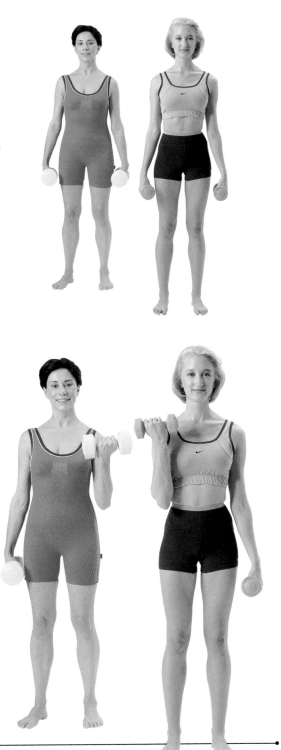

➲ Position one
Stand exactly as you did in the previous exercise, with your shoulders dropped well down and your head and neck free.

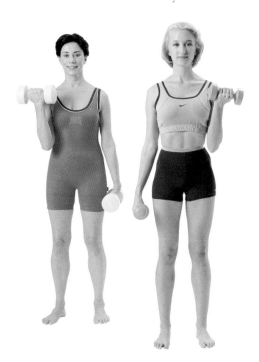

⌒ ➲ Positions two and three
Bend one arm at the elbow to raise the weight up towards your chest. As you lower it, start to raise the other arm. Alternate, 10 times on each side.

LUNGE

To exercise your triceps and biceps, stand in a lunge position, so as to prevent the strain of lifting the weight from going into the back. Keep the navel held in throughout, and check that you do not lift your shoulder as you take the arm back.

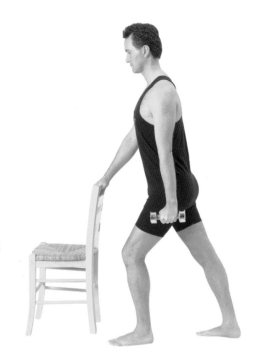

➲ Position one

Stand in a clear space with your right hand resting on a heavy piece of furniture. Place your left leg 30cm (1ft) in front of your right. Bend your left leg so you are leaning forwards in a lunge. Hold a weight in your left hand.

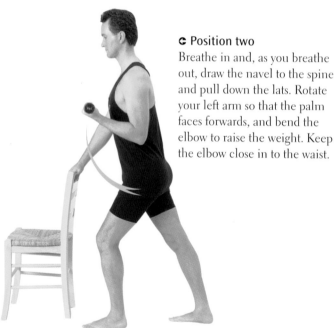

↺ Position two

Breathe in and, as you breathe out, draw the navel to the spine and pull down the lats. Rotate your left arm so that the palm faces forwards, and bend the elbow to raise the weight. Keep the elbow close in to the waist.

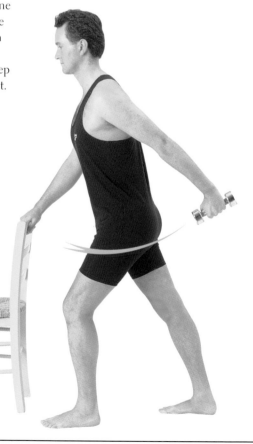

➲ Position three

Take your arm back, and repeat 10 times on each side.

Working the legs

REMEDIAL LEGS – ADVANCED

This is the last in this series of remedial leg exercises and combines a lift, a turning-out and a stretch. Always use one of the earlier remedial leg exercises (see pp. 72–73 and p. 98) as a warm-up.

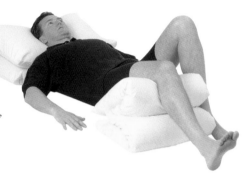

⟳ Position one
Lie on your back, with your head and shoulders supported on a large cushion, your right leg over another cushion, and your left leg bent with your foot on the floor.

⟲ Position two
Breathe in, and as you breathe out, draw in your abdominals and lift the right leg. When your leg is fully extended, point your foot, then flex it.

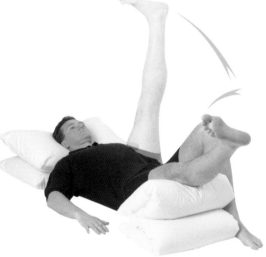

⟳ Position three
Turn out your leg from the hip. Breathe out as you lift it further across your body towards your left shoulder. This does not need to be a high lift – do not take the leg too far. Make sure your right hip remains on the floor.

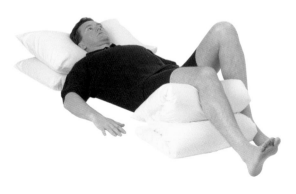

⟲ Position four
Take your leg back down to the cushion, turn it in, and lower your foot. Repeat slowly, 10 times on each leg.

Pliés

The plié is, of course, an exercise taken from ballet. It may look like a simple knee bend but it is, in fact, a complex movement when performed properly. Start with just the legs, concentrating on using the leg muscles correctly and keeping the back straight, and add the arm movements later.

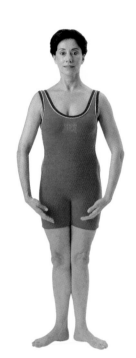

FIRST POSITION PLIÉS
⊃ Position one
Stand up straight with your thigh muscles pulled up, and a long spine. Keep your navel held in and squeeze the buttock muscles. Your neck should be long with the head held high. Curve your arms inwards. Bring your heels together with the toes pointed outwards.

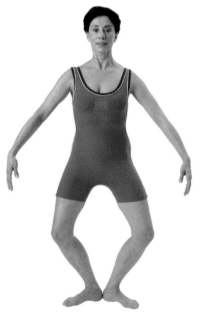

↶ Position two
Breathe in and, as you breathe out, bend your knees as much as you can without lifting the heels. As the knees bend they should remain over the feet. If they roll inwards, you are turning your feet out too much – try to narrow the angle. As you bend your knees, turn the thigh muscles out as if you are trying to make the inner thighs face the front. Also, as you bend your knees, your arms lift out to the sides.

STAY STRAIGHT

- *Never let the heels lift off the floor.*
- *Keep your spine straight at all times – don't arch, lean forwards or round the shoulders. If you do any of these, it may be because you are trying to turn the feet out too much.*
- *Keep the abdominal muscles held throughout.*
- *Don't let any tension creep into the neck or shoulders.*
- *The knees must always be in line with your feet.*

⊃ Position three
As you reach the limit of your knee bend, bring your arms forwards, still curved. Breathe in, and straighten your legs until you are in the starting position. Repeat 10 times.

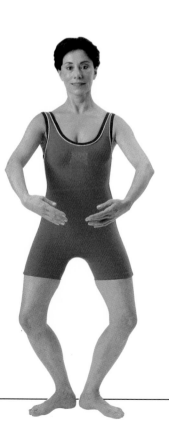

SECOND POSITION PLIÉS

↻ Position one

Stand with a long back and relaxed shoulders, this time with your feet about 30cm (18in) apart, and your toes pointing outwards in line with your knees. Keep your navel gently drawn in throughout the exercise. Hold your arms in a long curve, with fingers further apart than in the previous exercise.

➲ Position two

Begin to bend your knees, letting the back drop down, again imagining that the inner thigh and buttock muscles are trying to face the front. If your back leans or arches, or your knees roll in, adjust the position of your feet.

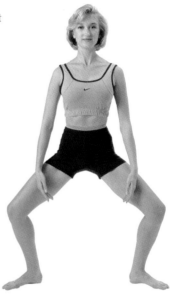

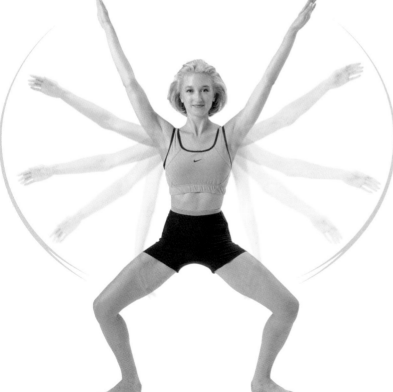

↻ Position three

As you bend your knees, start to raise your arms straight out to the sides, with the palms facing forwards.

When you reach the deepest bend, without lifting your heels off the floor, continue to raise your arms so that they point to the ceiling, but without lifting your shoulders. Then, as you straighten your legs, gently squeezing the thighs together, bring your arms gently back down to the starting position. Repeat 10 times.

Leg stretches

QUAD STRETCH

For this exercise you will need a strong, fairly high surface (such as a table or kitchen work surface), which will take your weight and allow your leg to reach the floor with a slight bend.

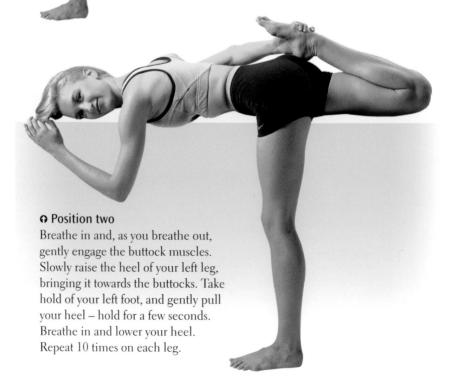

> ### TOO EASY?
>
> *If you can do this exercise easily, make it more difficult by placing a rolled-up towel under your leg, just above the knee. If you have difficulty reaching your heel with your hand, you can use a towel as a loop.*

↻ Position one

Lie face down on the side of a table or other surface with your right leg bent on the table, and your left foot flat on the floor. Rest the side of your face on the table and hold the edge of the surface loosely with your left hand.

↻ Position two

Breathe in and, as you breathe out, gently engage the buttock muscles. Slowly raise the heel of your left leg, bringing it towards the buttocks. Take hold of your left foot, and gently pull your heel – hold for a few seconds. Breathe in and lower your heel. Repeat 10 times on each leg.

HAMSTRING STRETCH

Here is a further stretch for the hamstring muscles, which need to be stretched regularly to counteract the effects of long-term sitting.

➲ Position one

Sit on a chair with your knees bent at a 90° angle. Stretch out the left leg and place a thick book under the heel. Rest both hands gently on the right leg just above the knee.

Take a deep breath in and, breathing out, stretch the whole spine up, leaning slightly back and looking upwards. Keep the spine, neck and head in alignment.

↶ ➲ Positions two and three

With the back, neck and head still in line, breathe out and lean forwards, rotating around the axis of the hip to stretch over the right leg until you feel a stretch in the hamstring. Hold the stretch briefly. Breathe in, and then breathe out as you curl the torso forwards over the leg. In a ripple starting from the pelvis, and running straight up the spine, curl up until you reach the starting position. Repeat 10 times for each leg.

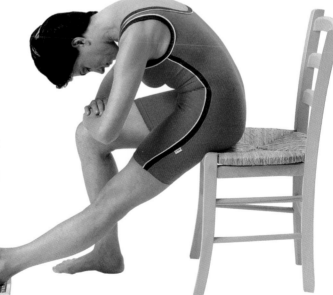

Advanced abdominals

Pilates technique teaches you to hold your stomach muscles lightly but firmly as a matter of course – and this advanced oblique and side stretch will certainly test how strong these muscles have become. If this is too much of a strain, you will see them bulge out, putting undue pressure on the stomach muscles and the back. If they do this, stop immediately. Take it gently and do only one or two repetitions to start. Remember in Pilates, strain and pain are not the aim.

TAKE CARE!

This is a powerful exercise. Do not hold the position for too long and stop immediately if there is any strain. Check your neck and shoulders for tension as well as your back and abdominals. You can also try this one lying against a wall to help you maintain the correct position.

SIDE STRETCHES
↺ Position one

Lie on your left side with your lower leg bent and your upper leg stretched out fully. Hook your top foot under a piece of furniture or ask someone to hold it in place. Your right arm should be stretched along your body, while your left arm is bent at the elbow, with your hand resting lightly on your shoulder.

↻ Position two

Breathe in deeply. As you breathe out, feel your upper body lengthen and slowly lift from the floor in one piece. Keep your back straight and your abdominal muscles pulled in. Breathe in and lower. Repeat, building up to 10 times each side.

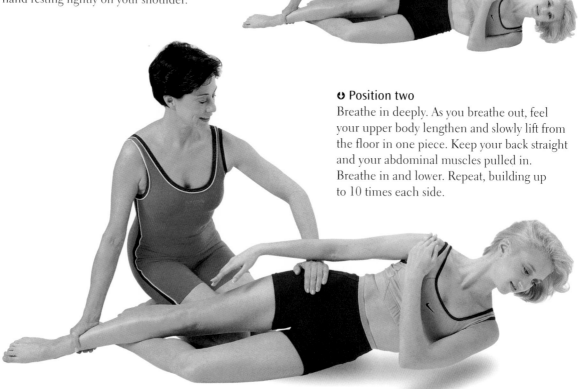

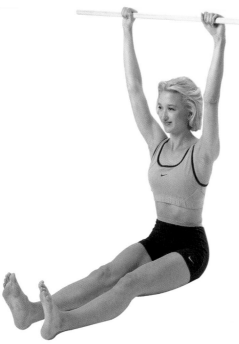

ULTIMATE ABDOMINALS
↻ Position one

Sit on the floor with your legs straight out in front of you, and your feet slightly apart and flexed. Sit up very tall with relaxed shoulders. Hold a pole or a rolled-up towel in your hands, and lift your arms straight above your head without lifting your shoulders.

↷ Position two

Breathe in and, as you breathe out, draw the navel to the spine and start to curl down through the back, gradually lowering your arms.

Continue the curl down until the pole reaches your thighs and the curve extends through the spine and into the neck, so that your head drops down slightly.

↪ Position three

Breathe in and, as you breathe out, hold the position of the body but raise the pole as far as you can, if possible bringing your arms back up to your head. Return the pole to the thighs, breathe in, and sit up into position one. Repeat up to 4 times.

Final muscle release

These are the final stages of the cushion squeezes – and hard work! If you are tired by this point, do one of the cushion squeezes from level one or two (see pp. 76 or 101).

KNEE SQUEEZE

The effort here should not go into the neck and shoulders – make sure that they stay relaxed throughout this exercise.

⊃ Position one
Lie flat on your back with your knees raised and a hard cushion between them. Place your hands by your sides.

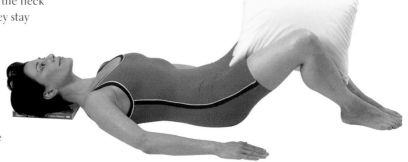

↺ Position two
Breathe in and, as you breathe out, draw the navel to the spine and squeeze the cushion between the knees.

⊃ Position three
As you squeeze, roll your head up, and your shoulders too, if possible, while lifting your arms slightly.
    Breathe in and roll down slowly. Repeat up to 5 times.

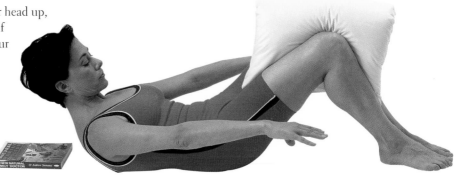

CUSHION SQUEEZE WITH FEET

Again, check that the effort here is made by the legs and the abdominal muscles. Don't let it creep into the back, neck or shoulders.

↻ **Position one**
Lie flat on your back with your legs stretched out in front of you. Place your arms by your sides.

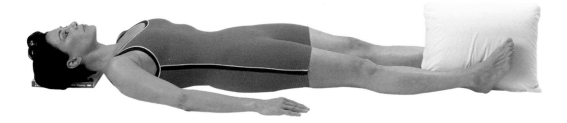

↻ **Position two**
Breathe in and, as you breathe out, draw the navel to the spine and squeeze the cushion between your feet.

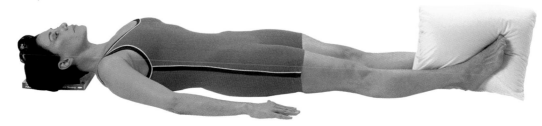

↻ **Position three**
If you can, try to raise your head up from the floor as you squeeze the cushion. Breathe in to roll down. Repeat up to 5 times.

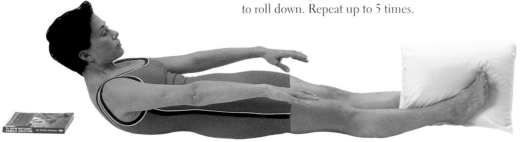

Appendix

Golden rules of Pilates Technique

- *Always start with a warm-up.*
- *Take your time! The slower you do these exercises, the better.*
- *Stay in time with your breathing.*
- *Put all effort on the out-breath.*
- *Remember the mantra: breathe in and, as you breathe out, draw the navel to the spine.*
- *Keep checking your posture.*
- *Stay focused on what your body is doing.*
- *Build up abdominal strength slowly. If your abdominals bulge out during an exercise, stop.*
- *Move your arms and shoulders from the lats and trapezius, not the shoulders themselves.*
- *Follow the instructions for the number of repetitions. Quality, not quantity, is what matters.*
- *Perform Pilates exercises regularly, ideally every other day.*
- *Don't give up – grace and poise can be yours if you persevere.*

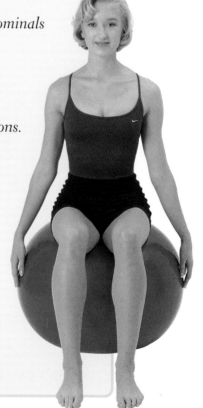

Glossary

MUSCLE GROUPS AND HOW THEY HELP

The **Abdominal** group of muscles extends much further than most people realise, running all the way down to the pubic bone. The main muscle (Rectus abdominis) runs all the way down the front of the abdomen and is the one constantly referred to in the Pilates mantra of 'draw the navel to the spine'.

- ➲ The **Oblique abdominals** help you move from side to side.
- ➲ The **Rectus abdominals** bends you forwards.
- ➲ The **Transverse abdominals** hold in the organs, for example when you draw the navel to the spine, they hold in the abdominal organs.
- ➲ The **Pelvic floor** is the group of muscles that support and contain the lower organs (womb, bladder and bowel).
- ➲ The **Biceps muscles** at the front of the upper arms bend and flex the arms and turn the hands outwards.
- ➲ The **Deltoid muscles** on top of the shoulders and upper arms move the arms up and down, and extend them out to the sides.
- ➲ The **Gluteus maximus** is the main muscle in the buttocks, and is vital for good posture. It is part of the Pilates 'girdle of strength' and should be firm. Ideally, it works in sychronicity with other muscles to create good posture.
- ➲ The **hamstrings** run down the backs of the thighs. They bend the knee and support the pelvis. If they are tight, they can put a strain on the lower back.
- ➲ The **Latissimus dorsi**, or 'lats', are the muscles running from below the shoulder blades to the pelvis. They support the shoulder blades and keep them down. Pulling down the 'lats' helps to lengthen the spine and initiate good arm movements and posture.

- ➲ The **Quadriceps**, or 'quads', are the muscles along the front of the thighs. They help you bend or extend your leg, lift it forwards, flex the thigh and bend your knees when you walk.
- ➲ The **Sternum**, also known as the breastbone, joins the ribs together.
- ➲ The **Trapezius muscle** runs from the shoulders upwards through the back of the neck. It supports the upper back and arms. It is often very tight, owing to stress accumulated there. In Pilates technique, the trapezius and the lats are generally used together to take the strain off the shoulders.
- ➲ The **Triceps muscles** at the back of the upper arms help the arms to straighten out.

OTHER TERMS

- ➲ **In one piece**, for example 'move the arms backwards in one piece', means move your body in one smooth, graceful movement.
- ➲ **Draw the navel to the spine** is the phrase you will hear repeated most often in Pilates technique. Make sure the effort is on the out-breath, and as you do this, you will feel your pelvis push forwards, your buttocks tuck in and tighten, your pelvic floor tighten up (if you are a woman) and the air push out from your lungs. Your posture will automatically improve. If you are not sure that you are doing it correctly, stand sideways to a mirror and practise, noticing the difference in your posture.
- ➲ **With a long neck**: if your shoulders are down, your spine is aligned and your posture correct, then your neck will be naturally elongated.
- ➲ **With a neutral spine** refers to the natural curve of the lumbar spine, neither too arched nor too flat.

Resources & useful addresses

Alan Herdman Studios
17 Homer Row
London
W1H 1HU
Tel: 020 7723 9953
Website: www.alanherdmanpilates.co.uk
Email: alan@alanherdmanpilates.co.uk

PILATES EQUIPMENT
Balanced Body
A Current Concepts Company
Suite 23
7500 14th Avenue
Sacramento
California 95820
USA
Tel: 001 916 454 2838
Fax: 001 916 454 3120
Website: www.balancedbody.com
Email: info@balancedbody.com

Acknowledgements

AUTHORS' ACKNOWLEDGEMENTS
Alan Herdman and Anna Selby would like
to thank Karon Bosler, Noelyn George, and
Martin Gurnett for modelling, Richard Burns
for hair and makeup assistance, Honor Blackman
for writing the foreword, Robert Fitzgerald and
Carola Trier for being Alan's original teachers,
Shirley Hancock for physiotherapy advice, and
Balanced Body of California for supplying the
Pilates machines featured in the studio section.

PUBLISHER'S ACKNOWLEDGEMENTS
Gaia Books thanks Mary Warren and Sue Harper
for indexing and editorial assistance, Pip Morgan
for guidance, and Ann Crowther for on-the spot
matwork instruction.

Index